A Colour Atlas of

Cardiac Pathology

Geoffrey Farrer-Brown
MA, MB BChir, MD, MRC Path

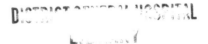
Wolfe Medical Publications Ltd
10 Earlham Street, London WC2

General Editor, Wolfe Medical Books
G Barry Carruthers, MD(Lond)

Other books in this series already published
A colour atlas of Haematological Cytology
A colour atlas of General Pathology
A colour atlas of Oro-Facial Diseases
A colour atlas of Ophthalmological Diagnosis
A colour atlas of Renal Diseases
A colour atlas of Venereology
A colour atlas of Dermatology
A colour atlas of Infectious Diseases
A colour atlas of Ear, Nose & Throat Diagnosis
A colour atlas of Rheumatology
A colour atlas of Microbiology
A colour atlas of Forensic Pathology
A colour atlas of Paediatrics
A colour atlas of Histology
A colour atlas of General Surgical Diagnosis
A colour atlas of Physical Signs in General Medicine
A colour atlas of Tropical Medicine & Parasitology

Further titles now in preparation
An atlas of Cardiology, ECGs and Chest X-Rays
A colour atlas of Standard Gynaecological Operations (6 volumes)
A colour atlas of Histological Staining Techniques
A colour atlas of Oral Anatomy
A colour atlas of Neuropathology
A colour atlas of Diabetes Mellitus
A colour atlas of the Pathology of Lymph Nodes
A colour atlas of Pedodontics
A colour atlas of Periodontology
A colour atlas of Gastro Intestinal Endoscopy
A colour atlas of Gastro Intestinal Pathology

Preface

This atlas is planned as a visual aid in Cardiac Pathology and not as a textbook. It is aimed at a mixed readership of senior clinical students, junior pathologists in training and other hospital staff interested in the subject. This may have resulted in sections which are too detailed for some readers and over-simplified for others.

In compiling this book the two major problems have been the availability of material and the limitation on selection due to restricted space. In general it is hoped that pictorially the topics are adequately covered although some omissions have been inevitable. For instance, aortic and great vessel disorders have only been included when associated with heart disease or when otherwise considered relevant. Common conditions have been described generally in greater detail than rare conditions, but the latter have been included when considered of educational value. A large section has been devoted to ischaemic heart disease in view of its frequency and importance in many parts of the world.

As selection must be personal I have on occasion indulged in special interests, acknowledging that this may alter the overall proportion of subjects. For instance, X-rays of the vasculature of the heart, which are not available collectively elsewhere, have been included in the hope that they will help in the understanding of myocardial infarction. Normal appearances are included where relevant.

To illustrate the macroscopical appearances both necropsy and museum specimens are included to give the student preparing for examinations a knowledge of the colour range in both types of material. As students of histopathology are normally provided only with haematoxylin and eosin stained sections the majority illustrated in this atlas have been stained by this technique and special staining methods have only been used to illustrate specific points.

Introductory texts to each chapter are brief, since students on questioning have indicated that they rarely read this part of the section. The legends describing the illustrations are of necessity also short, but when read in sequence are intended to describe salient points of each condition or disease.

To Jenny, James and Mark

Removal and examination of the heart

The techniques used for removal and examination of the heart vary according to the personal wishes of the pathologist but although there may be some variation in detail the basic procedure is usually similar. The following is a brief description of the technique used by the author but it should be remembered that it is modified if there is a need to demonstrate a particular abnormality, such as in congenital malformations of the heart.

REMOVAL OF THE HEART

First the pericardial cavity is examined after opening the anterior surface of the pericardium, usually by an inverted Y-shaped incision.

After careful external examination the following cuts are made to remove the heart. Blunt dissection is necessary before making some of the incisions.

1 The pulmonary artery and aorta are divided at the level of the transverse sinus. This is most easily done by first placing a finger through the transverse sinus behind the pulmonary and aortic trunks, as shown here, and then cutting across these vessels with a pair of scissors.

2 Cuts are made through first the left, as illustrated, and then the right pulmonary veins, close to the lungs. In each instance the heart is held aside to provide an adequate view and access to the vessels.
    1 = lung. 2 = liver.

3 The superior vena cava is divided as high as possible above the sino-atrial ring thus ensuring preservation of the sino-atrial node.

4 The inferior vena cava is cut just above the diaphragm, freeing the heart.

1

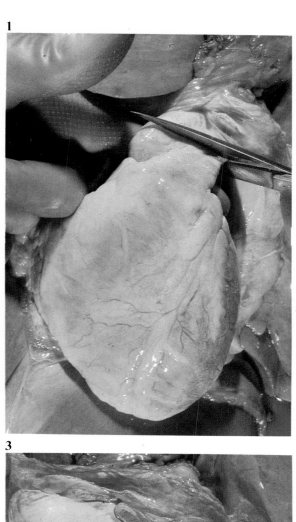

2

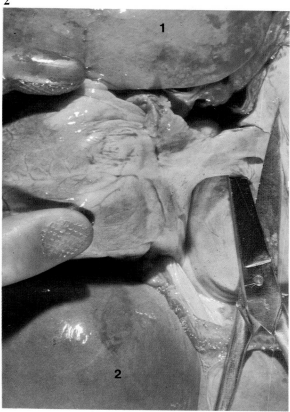

3

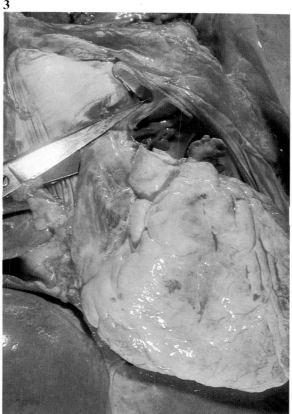

4

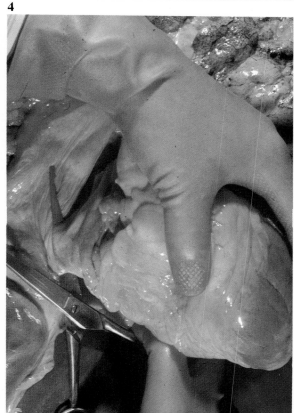

9

OPENING THE HEART

During the opening of the heart every structure must be inspected before cutting, and abnormal valves should be preserved intact.

Examination of the coronary arteries may be made while the heart is still intact or following its opening. The epicardial portions of the coronary arteries are best examined by making transverse cuts every 2mm, using a sharp scalpel. If calcification is present the vessel should be removed, fixed in formalin and then decalcified before cutting.

The incisions made by the author to open the chambers of the heart are as follows.

5 A cut is made across the ventricles about 3cm above the apex. It is convenient to keep the apical portion hinged by the epicardium posteriorly. When indicated, additional ventricular slices are cut as illustrated later.

5

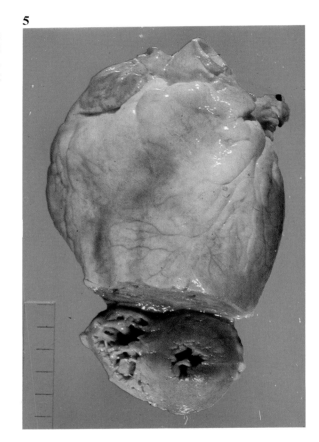

10 The left ventricle is opened by cutting down its lateral border to the apex.

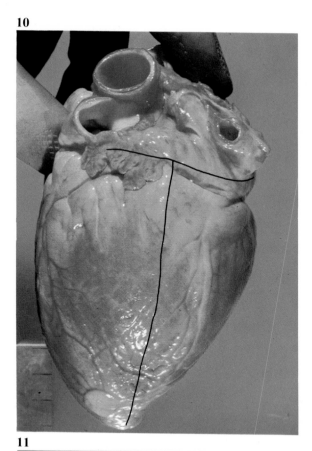

11 The outflow tract of the left ventricle is best viewed by cutting up the anterior wall close to the interventricular septum as far as the base of the auricular appendage when the cut is directed up into the aorta and across the aortic valve.

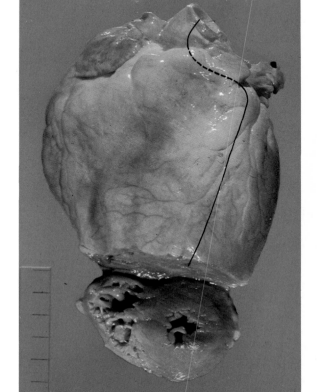

After completely examining the heart visually and removing blood from the chambers it should be weighed.

Special techniques such as examination of the conduction system (see figures **369** to **384**) or dissection of the ventricles for accurate weight assessment can then be carried out if indicated.

The normal adult heart

Illustrations of the normal adult heart are included in this section and where relevant in subsequent sections to allow comparison with pathological appearances.

12 Normal adult heart, anterior view Anterior view of a normal, 320g, adult male heart at necropsy. The orientation is different from the position of the heart in the body when the apex (1) points more forwards and to the left. In the base of this heart the first few centimetres of both the pulmonary artery (2) and aorta (3) are seen between the right (4) and left (5) atrial appendages. The division of the right (6) and left (7) ventricles is marked by the left anterior descending coronary artery (*arrow*) in the anterior longitudinal sulcus. The quantity of fat on the visceral pericardial surface varies, but tends to be greatest in obese patients.

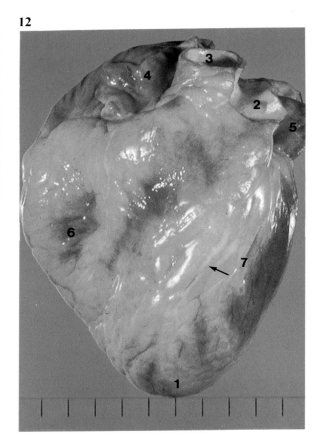

12

24 Normal adult heart, tricuspid valve The tricuspid valve of an adult heart is normally thin and translucent. The anterior leaflet (1), usually the largest, is on the right, the posterior (2), more variable in shape and size, on the left and the less distinct septal leaflet (3) in the middle. The chordae tendineae of these three leaflets are inserted respectively into a large anterior papillary muscle, a rather ill-defined posterior group of muscle columns, and into the wall of the interventricular septum.

24

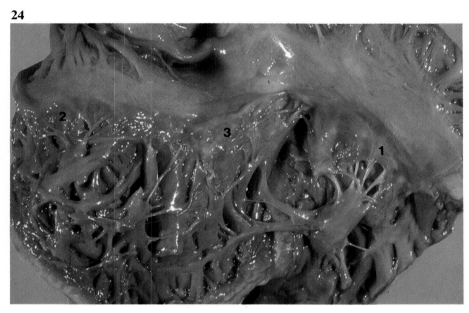

25 Normal adult heart, mitral valve An opened adult mitral valve. The valve is bicuspid with the anterior cusp on the left and the posterior cusp on the right. The anterior cusp, which separates the inflow and outflow tracts of the left ventricle, is continuous superiorly with the left and non-coronary cusps of the aortic valve, and is only attached to the myocardium at the commissures. The chordae tendineae of both leaflets are inserted into well-defined, prominent papillary muscles.

    1 = anterior cusp
    2 = posterior cusp

25

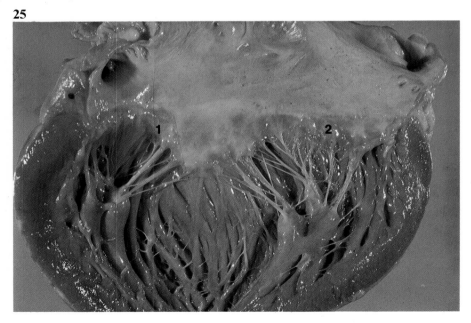

26 Cardiac muscle Myocardial fibres of the left ventricle of a 280g adult heart. The nuclei are centrally placed and oval or fusiform in shape. The capillaries alongside the muscle fibres are packed with red cells. (*H&E,* ×704)

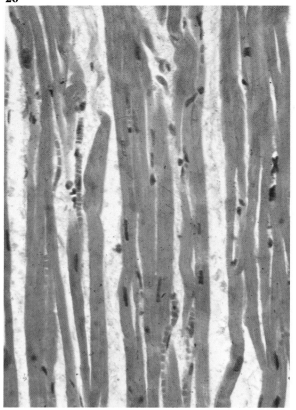

27 Cardiac muscle Cross striations of myocardial fibres are more clearly demonstrated using the phosphotungstic acid haematoxylin stain. (*PTAH,* ×1100)

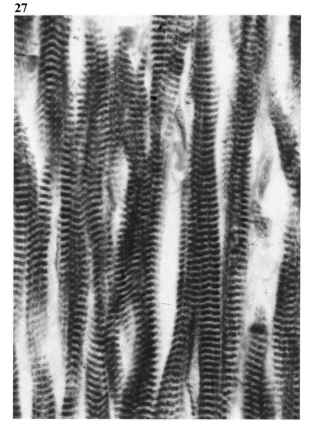

33 & 34 Atrial septal defect, secundum type Ostium secundum defects which occur in the region of the foramen ovale are variable in shape and size. Figure **33** shows a small defect while **34**, a museum specimen, illustrates a large defect with fenestration of the postero-superior rim. See **37** for a more extensively fenestrated defect. A small percentage of atrial septal defects are of the sinus venosus type when the septum primum forms to the right of the right pulmonary veins and is associated with imperfect incorporation of the sinus venosus into the right atrium, but this type is not illustrated.

33

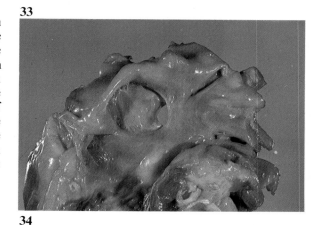

34

35 Atrial septal defect, secundum type, repaired The site of surgical closure, which was performed 5 years before death, of an ostium secundum, is indicated in this right atrium by a line of sutures embedded in white fibrous tissue, above the coronary sinus opening (*arrow*). The tricuspid valve is thickened as a result of the altered haemodynamics before repair of the defect. The heart was from a 26-year-old male. (*Museum specimen*)

35

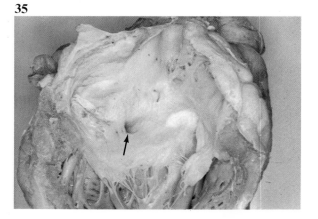

36 Atrial septal defect, primum type. An ostium primum defect which occurs below the fossa ovalis and involves the atrio-ventricular valves. This heart viewed from the left side shows a crescent-shaped upper border with the lower edge of the 3cm diameter defect extending down to involve the mitral valve, which has a cleft (*arrow*) in the anterior leaflet. (*Museum specimen*)

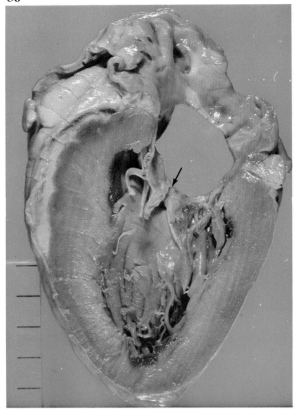

37 Atrial septal defect, persistent common atrio-ventricular canal An infant's heart with a more extensive ostium primum defect (1), or atrio-ventricularis communis. There is complete failure of fusion of the endocardial cushions (*arrow*) of the atrio-ventricular canal and consequent splitting of the mitral and tricuspid valves with an integral ventricular septal defect (2). In this heart there is also a separate fenestrated ostium secundum (3).

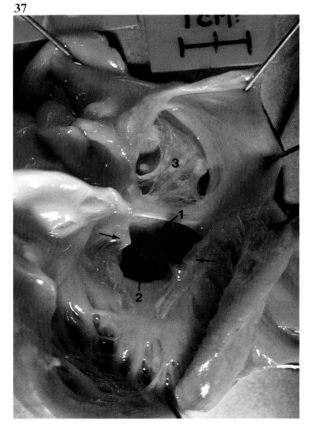

38 Ventricular septal defect A 'Fallot' type or 'high' defect (*arrow*) in the membranous part of the interventricular septum (see figures **42** and **43**). This view from the right ventricle shows the aortic valve (1) forming the roof of the defect.

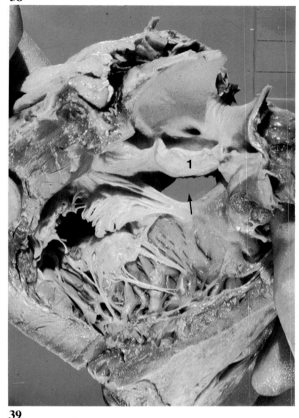

39 Ventricular septal defect Another type of defect of the membranous part of the interventricular septum, viewed from the right ventricle. This defect is infracristal in type, being situated postero-inferior to the crista supraventricularis. Alternatively it may be described as posterior to the papillary muscle of the conus (*arrow*). Uncommonly, defects may be supracristal or antero-superior to the crista supraventricularis.

40 Ventricular septal defect Defects also occur in the muscular interventricular septum, as illustrated here from the left side of the heart by a defect in the centre of the posterior part of the septum. This patient developed pulmonary hypertension as a complication of the defect. 1 = aortic valve. 2 = mitral valve. 3 = posterior papillary muscle.

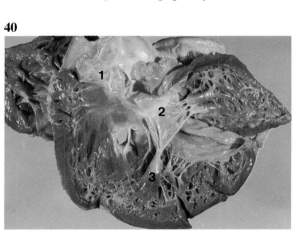

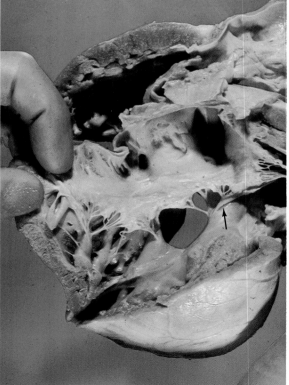

41 Single ventricle A single, or primitive, ventricle resulting from failure of the interventricular septum to develop. The mitral (1) and tricuspid (2) valves are both opening into the single ventricular cavity, the walls of which are hypertrophied. The papillary muscles are also abnormal. In this rare condition the aorta and pulmonary trunk are commonly transposed. (*Museum specimen*)

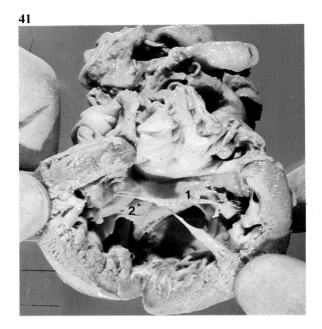

42 Fallot's tetralogy An infant's heart with Fallot's tetralogy. The anterior free wall of both ventricles has been cut away to show the aorta over-riding a ventricular septal defect (marked by a blue rod, see figures **38** and **43**) and thus communicating with both ventricular cavities. Another component of the tetralogy is a pulmonary stenosis which is due to infundibular obstruction (marked by a white rod) in this heart, but which can be valvar, or rarely supravalvar, in type, or combined. In addition, there is right ventricular hypertrophy. R = right. L = left.

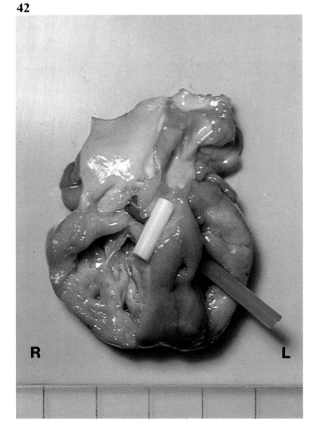

47 Congenital pulmonary valve atresia Superior view of an atretic pulmonary valve with fused cusps. This atresia may be associated with a 'Fallot' type ventricular septal defect, or the septum may be intact.

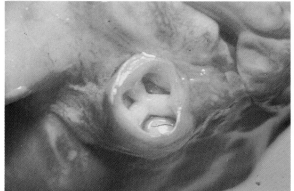

48 Congenital pulmonary valve stenosis Characteristic isolated dome-shaped, valvar, pulmonary stenosis (*arrow*) with a minute opening, in an infant's heart. Recent studies have suggested that left-sided heart disease with features similar to a hypertrophic cardiomyopathy may be associated with this defect in some patients. (*Museum specimen*)

    1 = pulmonary artery
    2 = pulmonary outflow tract

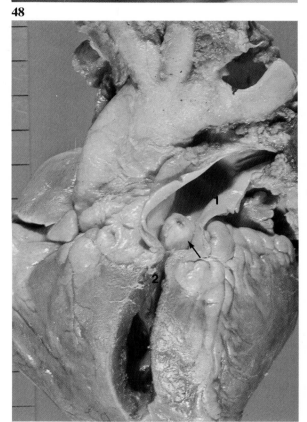

49 Congenital tricuspid valve atresia Superior view of an opened right atrium of an infant's heart with no tricuspid valve opening in the area ringed. In this heart there was also an atrial septal defect and a small ventricular septal defect through which pulmonary blood flow was maintained.

    1 = auricular appendage

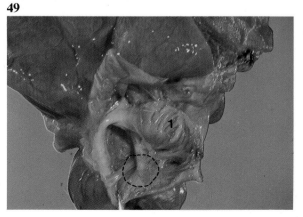

50 Congenital mitral valve stenosis An opened, thickened, stenotic mitral valve in an infant's heart. The valve leaflets have not become differentiated, there are no commisures and the chordae tendineae are short and thickened. The papillary muscles are also thickened but not illustrated. Other congenital heart abnormalities were associated with this mitral stenosis. (*Museum specimen*)

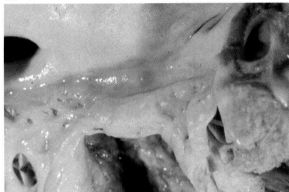

51 Subvalvar aortic valve stenosis The base of the heart viewed from below with a membranous subvalvar aortic stenosis (*arrow*) seen just above the anterior leaflet of the mitral valve. This type of stenosis can also be produced by a constricting ridge of fibrous tissue (see **319**). (*Museum specimen*)

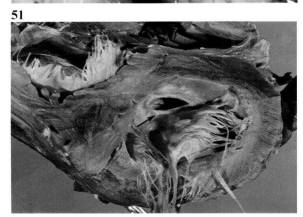

52 Congenital aortic valve stenosis Superior view of a stenotic aortic valve in an infant's heart. A black probe has been inserted into the orifice. This type of valve appears to consist of one cusp bending back on itself with one commissure (*arrow*). However, careful examination usually shows low raphes at the sites of the unformed commissures. Calcification is rare in this type of stenotic valve (see figure **62**). A second form of congenital aortic stenosis, which consists of a simple, dome-shaped valve with a central orifice, occurs but is not illustrated.

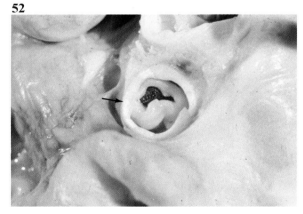

69 Petechial haemorrhages Small petechial haemorrhages scattered over the visceral pericardium of a dilated right auricle, occurring in a patient with thrombocytopenic purpura. Petechial haemorrhages may also be seen after death due to asphyxia.

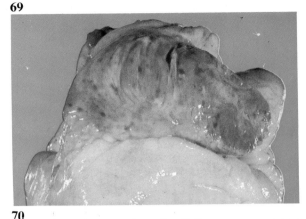

70 Haemopericardium This distended pericardial sac has been opened anteriorly to show the heart surrounded by a large quantity of blood. At necropsy the blood was coagulated but death had been caused by sudden entry of blood from a dissecting aneurysm of the thoracic aorta rupturing into the pericardial sac and producing acute cardiac tamponade. On the left is the distinctive appearance of blood distending the parietal pericardium (*arrow*). More commonly haemopericardium results from rupture of the wall following myocardial infarction (see **184**).

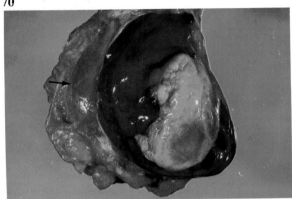

71 Fibrinous pericarditis The outer, or parietal, pericardium of the heart has been reflected upwards to demonstrate the characteristic 'shaggy' surface of a fibrinous pericarditis, described colloquially as a 'bread and butter' pericarditis.

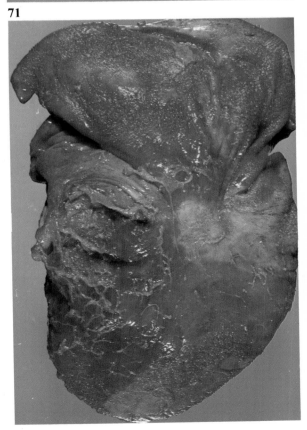

72 Suppurative pericarditis The pericardium has been reflected off the left ventricle but is adherent over the anterior wall of the right ventricle where a small incision has resulted in the extravasation of two beads of pus from a loculated suppurative pericarditis.

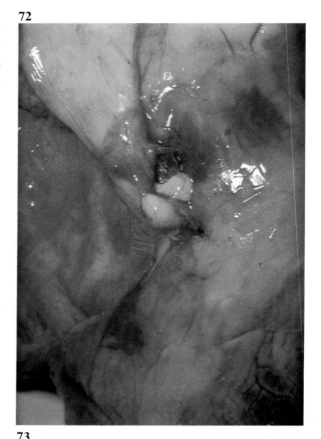

73 Suppurative pericarditis The parietal pericardium has been reflected off the anterior surface of the heart to show a diffuse suppurative pericarditis. The purulent exudate is best seen around the atrial appendages and overlying the pulmonary artery and aorta (*arrow*).

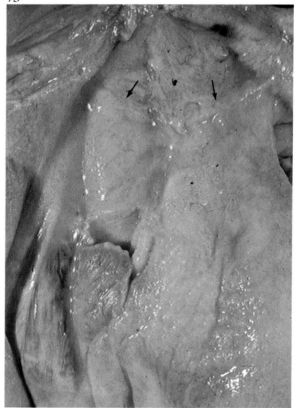

80 Rheumatoid pericarditis A rheumatoid pericardial lesion with an ill-defined central area of fibrinoid necrosis (1) surrounded by palisading histiocytes (*arrow*), lymphocytes and plasma cells. (*H&E,* × 280)

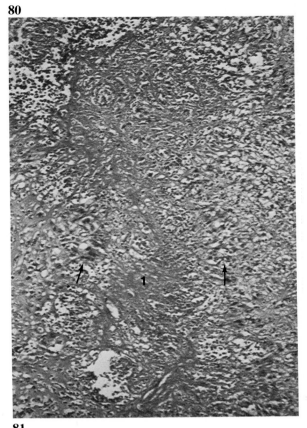

81 Constrictive pericarditis A densely fibrotic thickened pericardium. The outer myocardium is present on the left. The patient, a forty-year-old male, developed constrictive pericarditis following a Coxsackie B virus infection. (*H&E,* × 280)

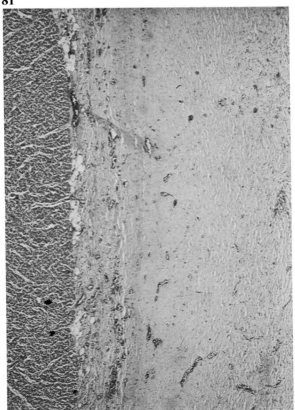

82 Calcified pericarditis Focal calcification is often present in a longstanding constrictive pericarditis. (*H&E,* ×176)

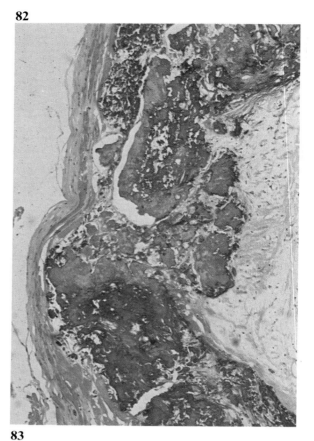

83 Carcinomatous pericarditis The posterior surface of a heart with nodules of secondary carcinoma of the breast scattered in the pericardium.

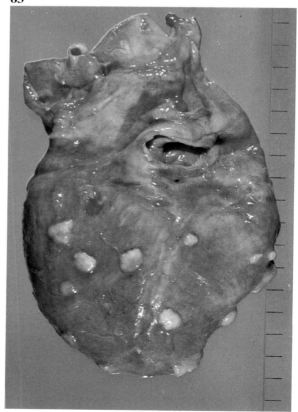

88 Normal pattern A necropsy arteriogram with both coronary arteries of a normal heart filled with radio-opaque medium. The courses of the individual main arteries are described in more detail in the next two figures. (See figure **87** for key to numbers.)

88

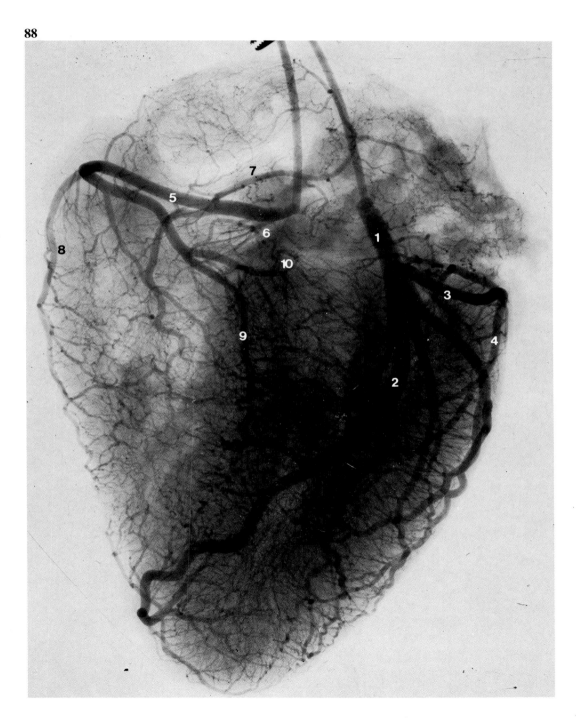

89 Right coronary artery, normal pattern Anterior x-ray of a normal right coronary artery (5) with the insertion of a short cannula indicating the position of the ostium. The main artery, coursing in the atrio-ventricular groove, soon gives off a conus branch (6) to the pulmonary outflow tract. In nearly a third of hearts the conus artery has a separate ostium in the aortic sinus. The sino-atrial node artery (7) is arising near the beginning of the main artery, an origin seen in 55 per cent of hearts. In 40 per cent, the sino-atrial node artery arises from the left circumflex artery (see figuré **90**), and in the remainder there is a dual blood supply from both the left and right coronary arteries. The main right coronary vessel then gives off a right marginal artery (8) and other smaller branches to the right ventricle and atrium. It is terminating here, as in over 90 per cent of hearts (see figures **93–94**), as the posterior descending coronary artery (9), which runs down in the posterior interventricular sulcus. The atrioventricular node artery arising from the right coronary artery at the origin of the posterior descending coronary artery is difficult to see in this x-ray. (× 1.2)

89

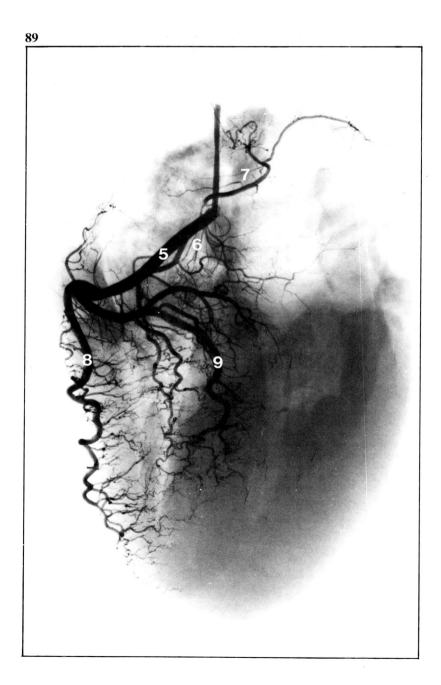

90 Left coronary artery, normal pattern Anterior x-ray of a normal left coronary artery (1) with a short cannula tied into the ostium situated behind the left cusp of the aortic valve. The main trunk, which varies in length, divides into the left anterior descending (2) and left circumflex arteries (3). The former artery passes down the anterior interventricular sulcus giving branches, one and sometimes two of which are often large vessels, to the anterior wall of the left ventricle. At the apex it usually curves round, as here, onto the posterior wall for a short distance, after which the terminal branches anastomose with the posterior descending artery. The left circumflex artery passes round in the left atrioventricular groove giving a left marginal branch (4) before terminating at a variable position on the lateral or posterior wall of the left ventricle. In this heart the sino-atrial node artery (7) is arising from the left circumflex artery (see figure **89**). (× 1)

90

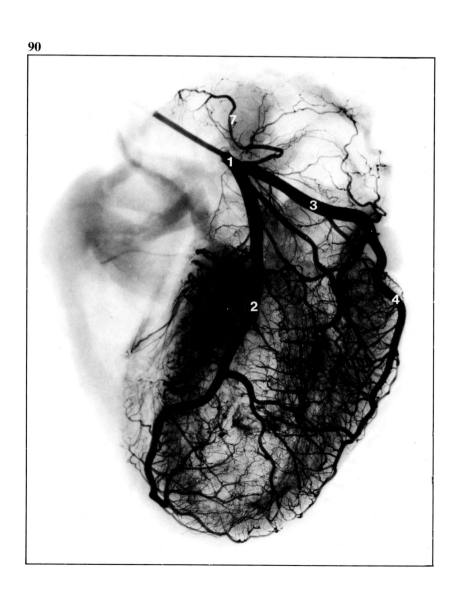

91 Coronary arteries, normal pattern An x-ray of
the coronary arteries in the base of the heart viewed
from above. The right coronary artery (1) is seen on
the left of the figure as it courses round in the right
atrioventricular groove. In this heart the left main
trunk (2) is very short and almost immediately
divides into the anterior descending (3) and left
circumflex arteries (4). The course of the latter vessel
in the left atrioventricular groove is clearly shown.
Only the first few centimetres of the anterior
descending artery are present but its first branches
to the anterior wall and the interventricular septum,
however, are shown.

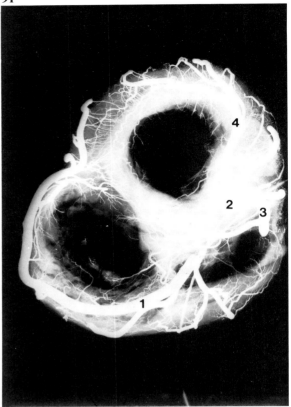

92 Coronary arteries, normal pattern A lateral x-ray
of the interventricular septum after removal of the
free walls of both the right and left ventricles. The
left anterior descending coronary artery (1) is seen
on the left as it passes down the anterior wall of the
heart in the interventricular sulcus. At the apex it is
curving round onto the posterior wall to anastomose with terminal branches of the posterior
descending artery (2), portions of which are present
on the right of the x-ray. Branches from the anterior
descending coronary artery supply the major part of
the interventricular septum.

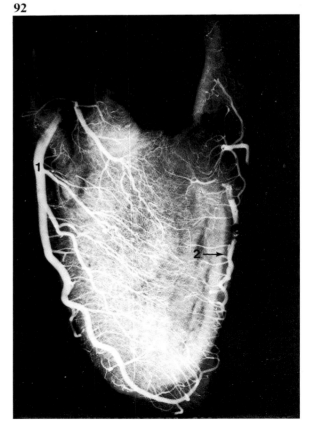

93 & 94 Coronary artery dominance The word 'dominance' is commonly used to indicate the artery that is supplying the major portion of the posterior wall. The author describes the pattern as right dominant when the right artery supplies the posterior walls of both ventricles (**93**), mid-dominant when the line of demarcation between the right coronary and left circumflex arteries is in line with the left edge of the interventricular septum (**94**), and left dominant in the small percentage of hearts in which the left circumflex artery supplies the whole of the posterior wall of the left ventricle, the posterior half of the interventricular septum and part of the posterior wall of the right ventricle. In general the sizes of the right coronary artery and left circumflex artery are in inverse relationship depending on which is the dominant vessel. This variation in domination is significant only in determining the area of myocardium that becomes ischaemic when either the right or the left circumflex coronary arteries are occluded. It should be remembered that in all hearts at least half of the left ventricular muscle bulk is supplied by the left coronary tree.

Yellow medium in right coronary artery tree.
Blue medium in left coronary artery tree.

93

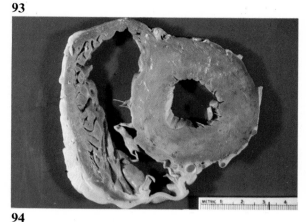

94

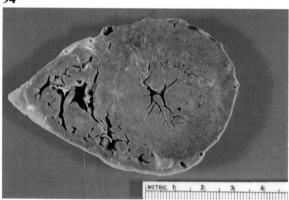

95 Myocardial vasculature, left ventricle The majority of the left ventricular myocardial wall is supplied by 'branching' type arteries which divide into smaller and smaller branches in a tree-like fashion as they pass through to supply the whole width of the myocardial wall. A typical example of this type of vessel is shown in this figure, an x-ray from the anterior wall of a left ventricle. (× 5)

96 Myocardial vasculature, left ventricle The second, but less numerous, variety of artery supplying the myocardial wall is known as a 'straight' type of vessel (*arrow*). They maintain their calibre as they pass through the myocardial wall and give off few branches until they terminate to supply the papillary muscles and columnae carneae. (× 4.5)

95

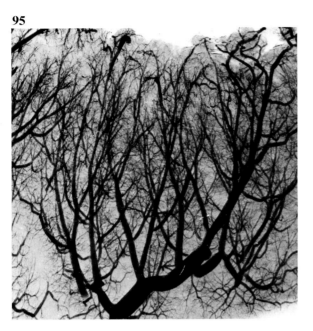

96

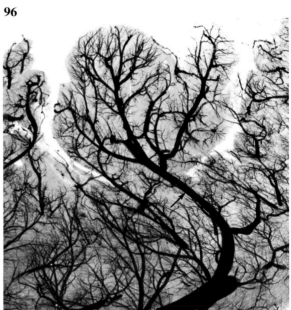

97 Myocardial vasculature The overall pattern of 'branching' and 'straight' type arteries supplying the left ventricular (1) free wall is shown in this x-ray of a midventricular slice of a normal heart. A similar vascular pattern is present in the right ventricular (2) free wall but is less obvious due to the smaller muscle bulk compared with the left. The main arteries in the middle of the interventricular septum (3) are branches of the anterior and posterior descending coronary arteries. (× 0.75)

97

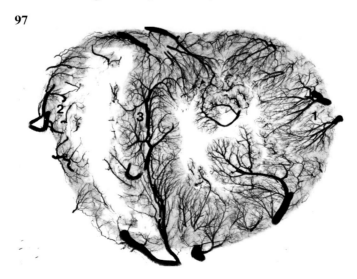

98 & 99 Myocardial vasculature, subendocardial
Knowledge of the vascular supply of the subendocardial zone of the left ventricle is important as it is
the most likely area to be damaged in myocardial
ischaemia. This figure illustrates the terminal
divisions of the 'branching' type arteries in the inner
part of the left ventricular wall, while **99** is a higher
magnification showing that these terminal branches
supply the myocardium right up to the endocardial
surface (1). (× 10.5, 15)

98

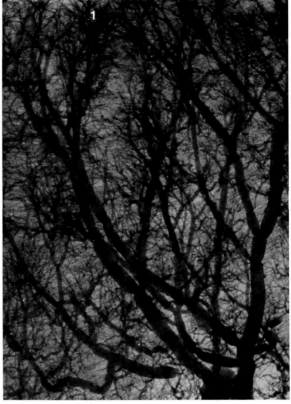

99

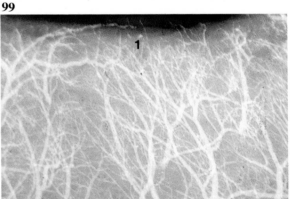

100 Myocardial vasculature, subendocardial The
author's definition of the subendocardial zone – the
innermost 2–3mm of the myocardium – does not
include the papillary muscles or columnae carneae.
This x-ray shows these muscle columns supplied by
'straight' type arteries while 'branching' type
arteries (*arrow*) supply the subendocardial zone
immediately adjacent to the columnae carneae.
(× 15)

100

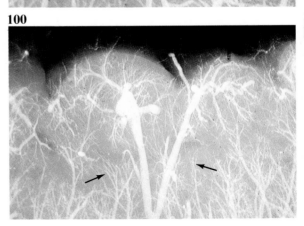

101 & 102 Myocardial vasculature, small arteries
The appearance of the terminal break-up of the
'branching' artery varies. It may be fan-shaped and
orientated in the direction of the artery (**101**) or the
branches may turn at right angles to the direction of
the main artery and then spread out before dividing
(**102**). These x-rays also show that the course of the
capillaries is determined by the direction of the
muscle bundles as these vessels run alongside the
muscle fibres. (× 90, × 50)

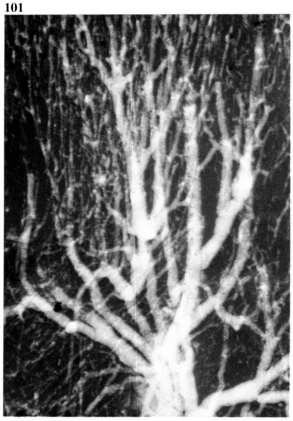

101

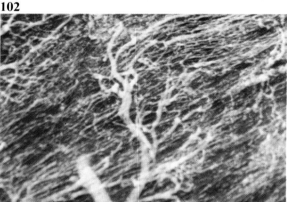

102

103 Myocardial vasculature, capillaries The
presence of capillaries alongside muscle fibres cut in
cross section is not usually obvious but filling these
vessels with radio-opaque medium (staining brown-
black) demonstrates their distribution (see next
two figures). (*H&E, × 550*)

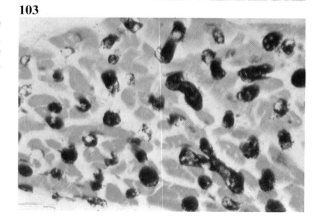

103

104 Myocardial vasculature, capillaries A 30μ thick histological section showing capillaries, filled with dark brown staining radio-opaque medium, running alongside muscle fibres. (*H&E,* × 1100)

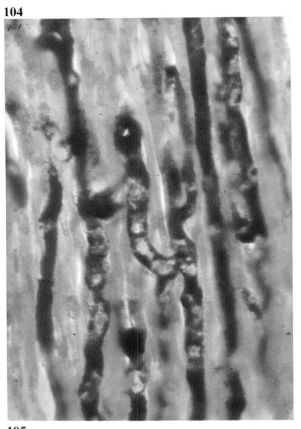

104

105 Myocardial vasculature High magnification of an x-ray of capillaries, with their fairly frequent cross communications, in the left ventricle wall. (× 1100)

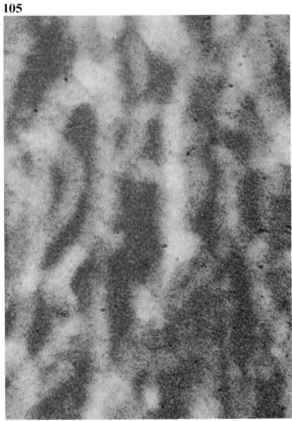

105

106 Myocardial vasculature, collateral arteries The existence of an extensive collateral system, which may be both extra and intramyocardial, is illustrated in this heart by the complete filling of both coronary trees, despite an atheromatous occlusion of the left anterior descending coronary artery (*arrow*). Severe atheroma is also present in the other main coronary arteries. The x-ray is a lateral, slightly oblique view. (× 0.78)

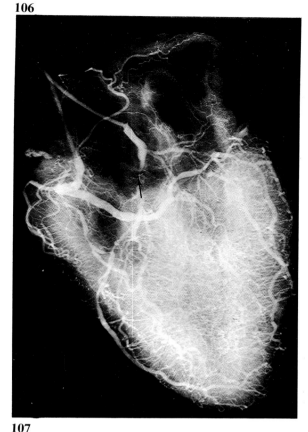

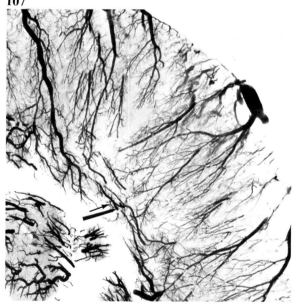

107 Myocardial vasculature, collateral arteries One of the main areas in which collateral arteries occur within the ventricular wall is in the subendocardial zone. This x-ray shows their circumferential course (*arrow*) compared with the normal radial direction of the 'branching' and 'straight' type arteries (see **95 & 96**). (× 4)

108 Myocardial vasculature, collateral arteries The collateral arteries in the myocardial wall allow important anastomotic communication between the anterior and posterior septal arteries. They are present at birth but only appear prominent in certain pathological conditions. Illustrated here, in close-up, are these vessels (*arrow*) in the heart of an infant who only survived two hours and died of the respiratory distress syndrome. (× 10)

108

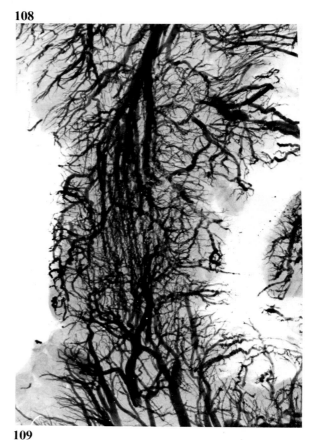

109 Myocardial vasculature, collateral arteries High magnification of a typical collateral artery in the interventricular septum of an adult heart with severe coronary artery atheroma. (× 9)

109

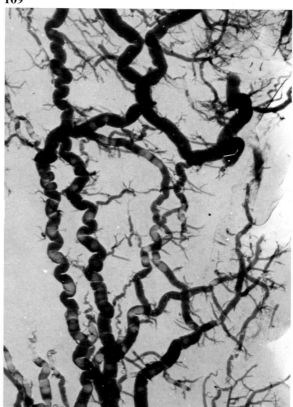

THE CARDIAC VEINS

110 The main extramural venous drainage of the heart is via a system of subepicardial veins that open into the coronary sinus, although a separate system of *anterior cardiac veins* (1) drains directly into the right atrium. The pattern of veins shows individual variation but a schematic representation is shown in this figure.

The *great cardiac vein* (2) forms at the apex or in the lower half of the anterior interventricular sulcus. It ascends to the proximal part of this sulcus and then curves sharply to the left to run in the left atrioventricular sulcus until it drains into the coronary sinus (3). This sinus, usually described as beginning at the site of the valve of Vieussens (4), courses posteriorly and to the right in the atrioventricular sulcus, finally opening into the right atrium below and medial to the orifice of the superior vena cava. The *posterior vein* (5) courses obliquely upwards across the posterior wall of the left ventricle opening into either the coronary sinus or the great cardiac vein. The *left marginal vein* (6) drains the lateral wall of the left ventricle and ends in the great cardiac vein. The *middle vein* (7) arises at the apex, courses up the posterior interventricular sulcus and usually drains into the distal portion of the coronary sinus. The *small cardiac vein* (8) is variable, but runs in the right atrioventricular groove ending at the opening of the coronary sinus, although it may drain into the middle cardiac vein. The *right marginal vein* (9) terminates in the small cardiac vein in approximately a third of patients, but is considered part of the anterior cardiac venous system.

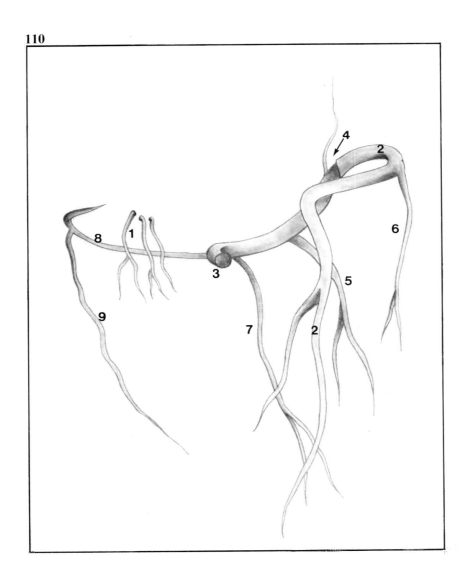

110

The following four figures illustrate the intra-mural component of the venous system of the heart.

111 Myocardial venous pattern, left ventricle X-ray of a 5mm transverse midventricular slice of a normal heart showing that the density of veins in the left ventricle is much greater than that of the arteries (see **97**). (× 0.75)
L = left
R = right

112 Myocardial venous pattern, left ventricle The pattern of myocardial veins in the left ventricle contrasts with the arterial branching system (see **95**) in that large drainage veins begin in the subendo-cardial zone and maintain a comparatively even calibre as they course towards the pericardium. (× 2.5)
1 = pericardium
2 = endocardium

113 Myocardial venous pattern, left ventricle In addition to the large drainage veins beginning in the subendocardial zone, similar, but smaller, veins drain the outer half of the wall. Close to the pericardial surface a small number of the main drainage veins converge to form a single vessel which drains into the large pericardial veins. Also in this subpericardial zone some of the small veins drain directly into the main pericardial veins. (× 5)
1 = pericardium

114 Myocardial venous pattern, interventricular septum The left half of the interventricular septum shows a vein pattern similar to the free wall of the left ventricle. Main drainage veins begin in the subendocardial zone (1) and course directly to enter the large central veins, running alongside the main septal arteries, near the middle of the septum (2). (× 8)

111

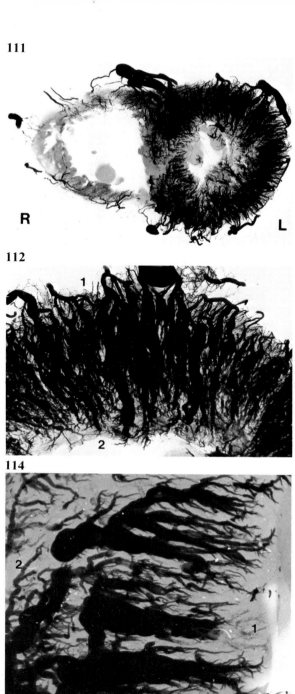

112

113

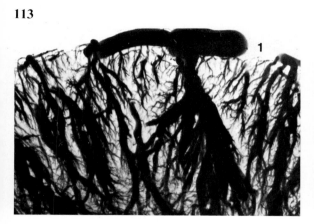

114

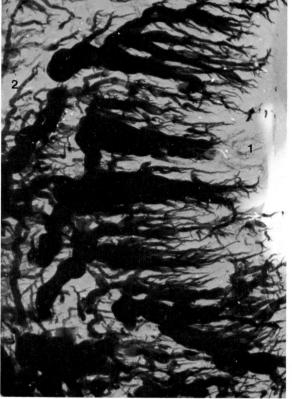

Coronary artery atheroma

In atheroma, or atherosclerosis, of the coronary arteries, the disease process is believed to begin focally in the intima, but at a later stage also affects the media and adventitia. The lesions appear to be due to a combination of degenerative and reactive proliferative processes. The development and appearances of atheromatous plaques is complex and in this section illustrations have been selected to show mainly extensive disease.

115 Coronary artery atheroma A left anterior descending coronary artery opened longitudinally to show the distribution of early atheromatous plaques around the openings of its branches (*arrow*). The heart was that of a 25-year-old male who died of multiple injuries.

116 Coronary artery atheroma A right coronary artery opened longitudinally to show an area of severe disease with atheromatous material exuding into the lumen. At the lower end of the plaque there is haemorrhage in the wall and an adjacent intimal tear.

115

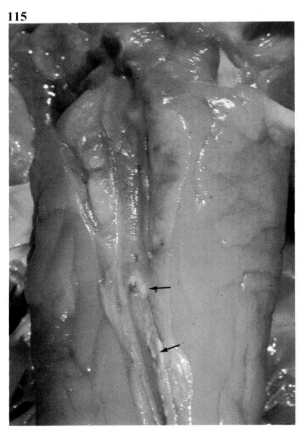

116

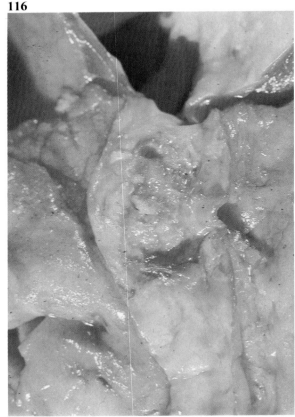

117 Coronary artery atheroma A right coronary artery opened to show occlusion by thrombus (*arrow*), superimposed on an atheromatous plaque 1.5cm from the ostia. Thrombi are the commonest cause of complete occlusion in patients dying of atheromatous coronary artery disease but reports of their incidence vary considerably. The author believes that they can be found in the majority of cases, more often in regional infarcts (see **157**) than laminar infarcts, and more often with increasing time of survival after the onset of ischaemia and with increasing size of infarcts.

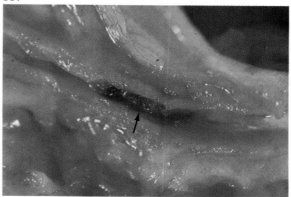

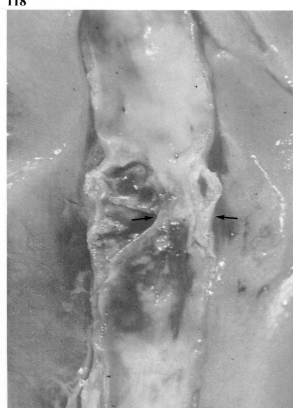

118 Coronary artery atheroma A coronary artery, opened longitudinally, to show partly organised thrombus incorporated into the wall on both sides of a narrow constriction (*arrow*) associated with a soft area of atheroma. The incorporation of mural thrombi may play an important role in the growth of atherosclerotic lesions.

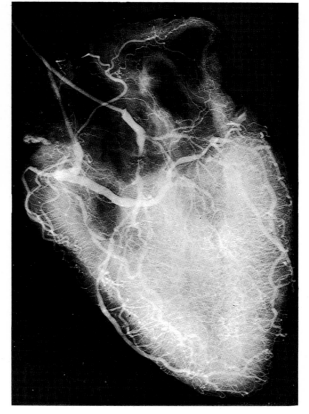

119 Coronary artery occlusion The commonest site of occlusion in atheromatous coronary artery disease is in the first 2cm of the left anterior descending coronary artery as illustrated in this lateral and slightly oblique x-ray of an injected heart of a man who died of myocardial infarction. The next commonest site of occlusion is the right coronary artery, classically as it bends at the lateral margin, followed by the proximal part of the left circumflex artery.

120–123 Coronary artery atheroma Assessment of the degree of stenosis is best appreciated by cutting the coronary arteries in cross-section. The shape and position of the remaining lumen in severely stenosed arteries is variable and, for example, may be eccentric or central and oval or round. The following four figures are cross-sections of coronary arteries with severe atheroma from hearts of patients who died of coronary artery disease.

120 A severely atheromatous coronary artery with much reduced lumen occluded by thrombus.

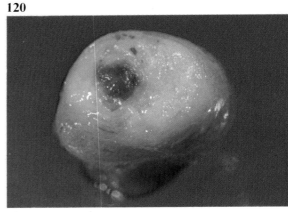

121 A left anterior descending coronary artery with the wall only moderately thickened by atheroma but the lumen occluded by thrombus.

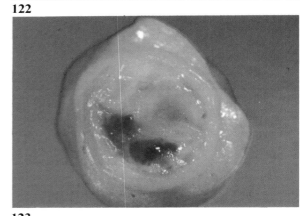

122 A severely atheromatous right coronary artery with a brown area on the left indicating the site of an old haemorrhage in the wall. The small eccentric lumen, in the lower part, is occluded by thrombus.

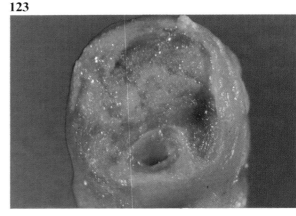

123 A coronary artery with the wall containing extensive soft atheromatous material and an area of old haemorrhage on the right. A small patent lumen is present in the lower part, for although the patient died from a myocardial infarct, no occluding thrombus was found.

124 Adult coronary artery The appearance and wall thickness of a coronary artery at necropsy is best appreciated following injection of radio-opaque material at systolic blood pressure. Illustrated here is a small right coronary artery from a normal heart of an East African, who had no evidence of coronary artery disease. It should be compared with a coronary artery with severe atheroma, from an Englishman's heart, in **128**. (*H&E*, ×8.8)

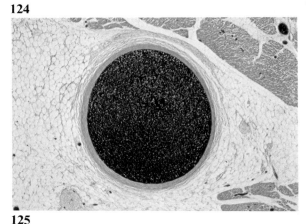

125 Adult coronary artery Close-up of the wall of the coronary artery illustrated in the previous figure. The intima (*arrow*) consists of a single layer of endothelial cells with an underlying longitudinal, thin, smooth muscle layer, while the media is composed of a thicker circular layer of smooth muscle. (*H&E*, ×550)

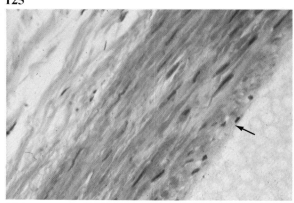

126 Adult coronary artery An elastic van Gieson stain of a normal adult coronary artery shows the internal elastic lamina (*arrow*) to be a straight black line lying beneath an intima unaffected by atheroma. Although this is the appearance of internal elastic lamina at systolic blood pressure during life it appears as a wavy line in most non-injected coronary arteries at necropsy (see next figure). (*EVG*, ×550)

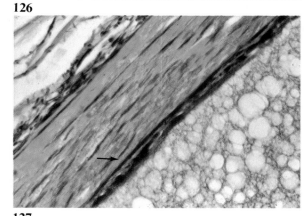

127 Adult coronary artery The wavy line appearance of the internal elastic lamina usually seen in a histological section of a coronary artery. The intima shows fibrous thickening with fragmented elastic tissue. This thickening may be the forerunner of atheroma and is seen focally in the arteries of infants. By adulthood the thickening is more diffuse and increases with age. (*EVG*, ×550)

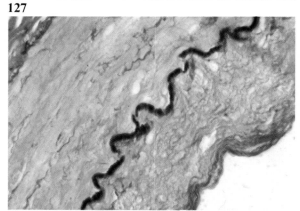

128 & 129 Coronary artery atheroma Cross-section of a coronary artery severely affected by atheroma stained by haematoxylin and eosin (**128**) and Martius scarlet blue (MSB) (**129**). The lumen, markedly reduced by atheroma, was terminally occluded by thrombus, but in preparation of the sections this has shrunk away from the intima. The histological features that may be present in varying proportion in any severely diseased artery, associated with destruction of the normal architecture of the wall, are: Lipid and foam cells, fibrin, cholesterol crystals, chronic inflammatory cell infiltrate, increased vascularisation, haemorrhage, thrombus, fibrosis, necrosis and calcification. These components are illustrated in **130–139**. (× 8.8 × 8.8)

128

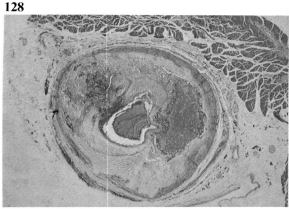

129

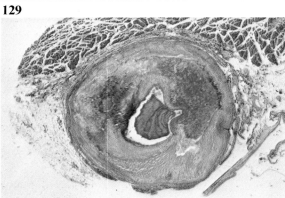

130 & 131 Coronary artery atheroma A 'soft' area of atheroma consisting of numerous foam cells surrounded by recent and previous haemorrhage. Scattered cholesterol crystal spaces are also present. Some of the different components are difficult to distinguish in the H&E section (**130**) but are more easily seen in **131**, an MSB stain. In this latter section fibrin is red staining, erythocytes yellow, foam cells pale pink and fibrous tissue blue. (× 8.8, × 8.8)

1 = lumen
2 = fibrous tissue

130

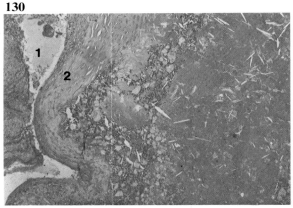

131

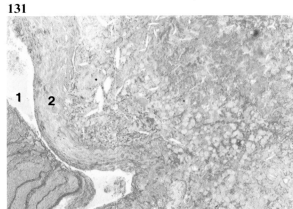

132 Coronary artery atheroma High magnification of foam cells (*arrow*) lying amongst erythrocytes and fibrin as seen on an H&E section. (*H&E*, ×352)

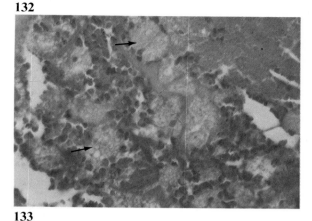

133 Coronary artery atheroma The appearance of the foamy macrophages with their granular cytoplasm (*arrow*), is more clearly seen in an MSB stain. Erythrocytes = yellow. Fibrin = bright red. (×352)

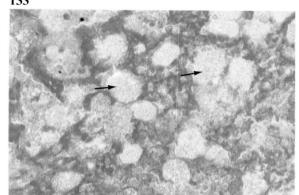

134 & 135 Coronary artery atheroma Elongated, oval or needle-like spaces (*arrow*) caused by the presence of cholesterol crystals. The cholesterol, however, has been dissolved during processing of the artery prior to sectioning so that only these characteristic empty spaces are seen. Figure **134** illustrates them in a section stained by MSB, while **135**, an H&E section, shows a foreign body giant cell reaction (*arrow*) to cholesterol. (×352, ×220)

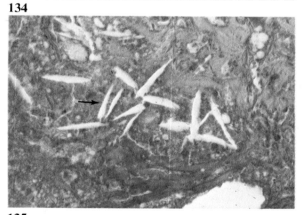

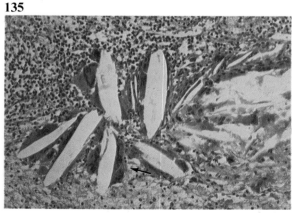

136 Coronary artery atheroma Chronic inflammatory cell infiltrate present in fibrous atheromatous tissue. Erythrocytes = yellow. (*MSB*, × 352)

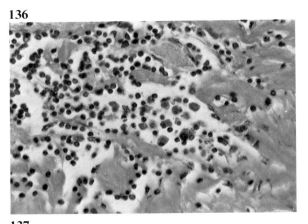

137 Coronary artery atheroma Calcification (*arrow*) within the deeper intimal fibrous component of an atheromatous plaque. In approximately half the patients with ischaemic heart disease the calcification is sufficiently extensive to be seen radiologically. (*H&E*, × 140)

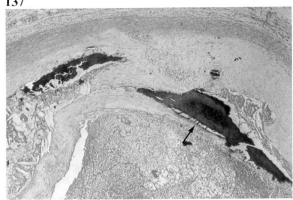

138 Coronary artery atheroma Increased vascularisation of the wall of an artery with severe atheroma. The media is seen on the right and the lumen on the left. (*H&E*, × 88)

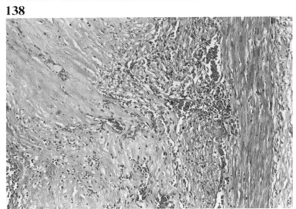

139 Coronary artery atheroma In severely diseased atheromatous arteries there is often adventitial fibrosis and an inflammatory cell infiltrate which tends to be perivascular in the adventitia. (See also figure **144**.) Fibrous tissue is blue (*MSB*, × 88)

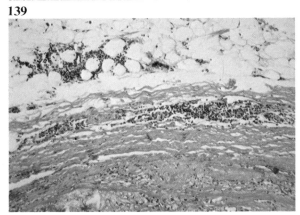

140 Coronary artery atheroma Close up of an intimal rupture (*arrow*) in a coronary artery with severe atheroma. This type of tear, usually overlying an area of 'soft' atheromatous tissue, may be an important initiating factor in thrombosis. However, care must be taken to exclude the possibility that the tear is an artefact occurring during processing and sectioning of the artery. (*H&E,* ×22)

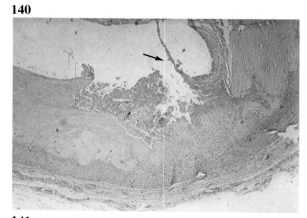

141 Coronary artery atheroma High magnification of an intimal tear in a coronary artery with severe atheroma. Haemorrhage (1), present in the wall of the artery, is in continuity with thrombus (2) occluding the lumen. A torn-off portion of intima is seen on the right (*arrow*), lying in the thrombus at a right angle to the wall. (*H&E,* ×88)

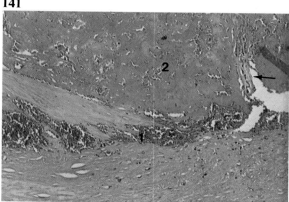

142 & 143 Coronary artery atheroma Two coronary arteries occluded by recently formed thrombus adherent to the atheromatous wall. The lumen in figure **142** is oval and central, while in figure **143** it is smaller and eccentric. (*H&E,* ×22, ×22)

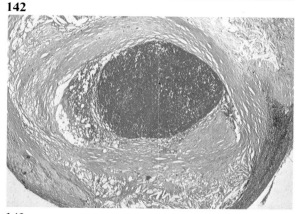

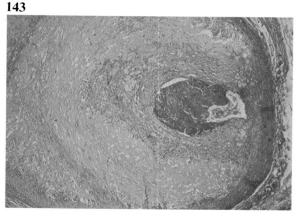

144 & 145 Coronary artery atheroma Partial organisation of the thrombus occluding this coronary artery has occurred so that only a wedge-shaped area of red thrombus remains. (× 8.8)

Figure **145** shows detail of the capillary vessels and fibroblasts in the area of organisation. (× 88)

144

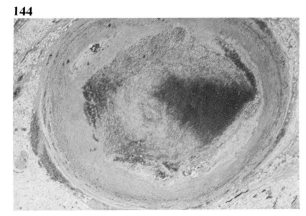

145

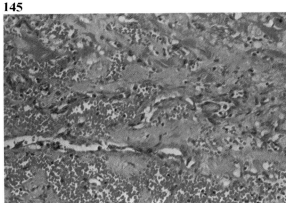

146 Coronary artery atheroma The lumen of this atheromatous coronary artery is occluded by fibrous tissue which resulted from organisation of occluding thrombus. (*H&E*, × 22)

146

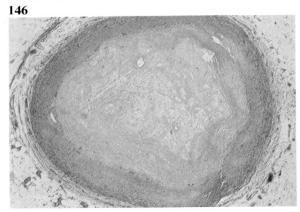

147 Coronary artery atheroma Following complete occlusion of a coronary artery recanalisation may occur with the formation of small channels (1), as in the high magnification of the centre of this artery. Increased vascularisation of the inner intima and a chronic inflammatory cell infiltrate are also present. (*H&E*, × 55)

147

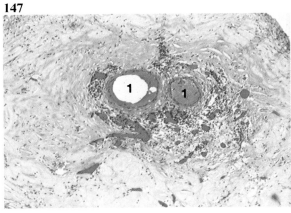

148 & 149 Coronary artery emboli Occlusion of the main coronary arteries by emboli is uncommon, but may result from endocardial thrombi, or vegetations, on the left side of the heart. Recanalisation can occur with the formation of either small or large channels as illustrated. Neither of these arteries, which are from the hearts of East Africans, are affected by atheroma. (*EVG*, ×22, ×22)

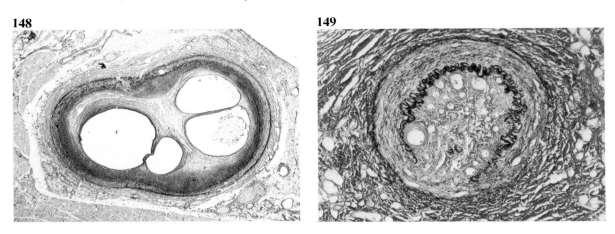

150–153 Myocardial small artery emboli The following four figures show varying appearances of small arteries in the myocardium that have been occluded by thrombotic emboli. The first vessel has been recently occluded while the thrombus in the second is partially organised. Organisation of the thrombus in the third and fourth arteries is complete with recanalisation by small channels. (×88, ×140, ×88, ×88)

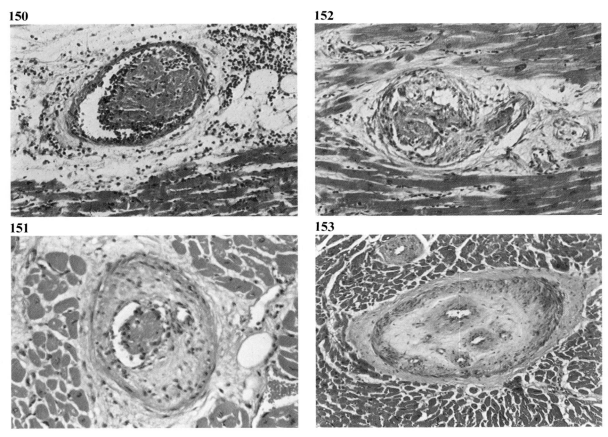

Myocardial infarction

Myocardial infarction results from ischaemia of the myocardium which, in the vast majority of hearts, is due to atheromatous coronary artery disease. Emboli, syphilitic ostial stenosis, isolated aortic stenosis, aneurysms, trauma and surgery, arteritis and congenital abnormalities are uncommon causes of insufficient coronary artery flow. A sequence of gross and microscopical appearances of myocardial infarction are illustrated in the following section.

154 Myocardial infarct, anterior An apical and anterior wall myocardial infarct (*arrow*) which resulted from occlusion of the left anterior descending coronary artery. In addition there is a generalised fibrinous pericarditis.

155 Myocardial infarct, anterior Transverse ventricular slices have been cut from the apex of the heart illustrated in the previous figure. The infarct involves the whole of the apical slice, but in the upper slice infarction is confined to the anterior wall of the left ventricle and the anterior half of the interventricular septum. Note also the endocardial thrombus.

154

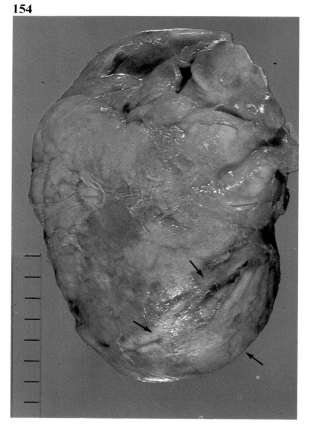

155

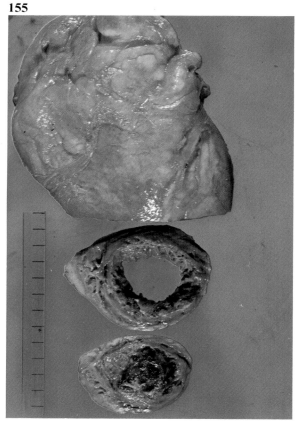

156 Myocardial infarct, posterior Posterior view of a heart with the upper two-thirds of the posterior wall of the left ventricle appearing haemorrhagic. The infarct resulted from occlusion of the right coronary artery, in a heart with a right dominant pattern (see **93**), six days before death. A pericardial patch is also present (see **74**).

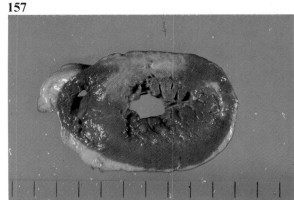

157 Myocardial infarct, regional type An infarct involving the full width of the posterior left ventricular wall and posterior half of the interventricular septum in the region of supply of the right coronary artery. This regional type of infarct, which is the more common, contrasts with the laminar, or subendocardial, type illustrated in the next figure.

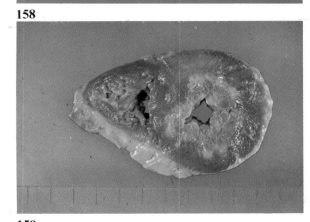

158 Myocardial infarct, laminar type A circumferential laminar infarct involving the majority of the inner half of the left ventricular free wall and the left half of the interventricular septum. This type of infarction is seen usually in hearts with severe atheroma of all the main arteries and may occur in association with regional infarcts (see **200**).

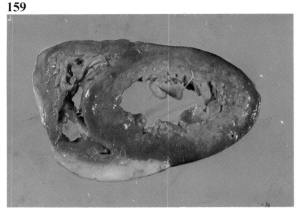

159 Myocardial infarct Pallor is the initial gross change that can be seen in an area of infarction and is usually apparent about 12–15 hours after the onset of ischaemia. This transverse ventricular slice shows extensive areas of pallor in the left ventricular wall following occlusion of the main trunk of the left coronary artery in a heart with a left dominant pattern (see **93**).

160 Myocardial infarct By about 36 hours the area of pallor becomes surrounded by a haemorrhagic zone, as in the posterior wall of the left ventricle of this heart.

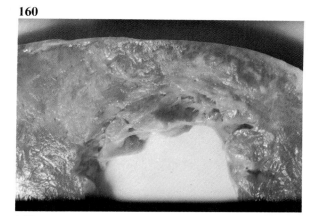

161 Myocardial infarct The haemorrhagic zone of the infarct illustrated in the previous figure is more clearly seen after photographing the specimen under water.

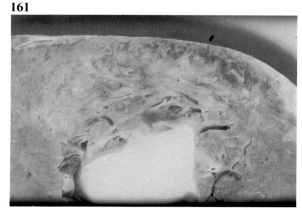

162 Myocardial infarct The centre of the infarct becomes more opaque and the haemorrhagic border more distinct after approximately 3–4 days.

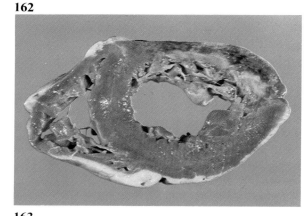

163 Myocardial infarct An area of ischaemic myocardium may enlarge, possibly due to extension of coronary artery thrombosis, some time after the initial infarction. In this transverse ventricular slice the infarcted area has extended from the initially damaged anterior wall (1) into the anterior half of the interventricular septum (2). Subendocardial fibrosis (3) and thinning of the lateral wall indicates a previous area of myocardial ischaemia.

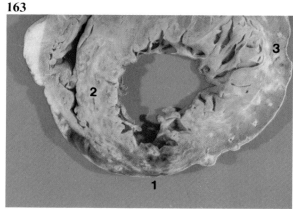

164 Myocardial infarct Haemorrhage may occur as seen in the centre of this 4-day-old infarct in the posterior wall of the left ventricle.

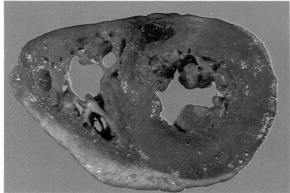

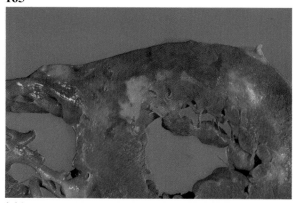

165 Myocardial infarct As the centre of the infarct becomes necrotic it appears yellow and structure-less, as illustrated in the posterior wall of the left ventricle of this transverse ventricular slice. Note that by this stage the haemorrhagic margin has become prominent.

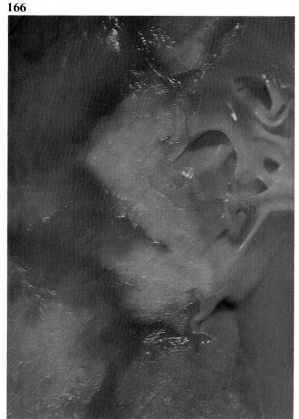

166 Myocardial infarct Detail of the area of infarction illustrated in the previous figure. *Myomalacia cordis,* literally softening of the heart muscle, is sometimes applied to an infarct at this stage.

167 Myocardial infarct The lateral wall of the left ventricle cut longitudinally to show an infarct (*arrow*) of similar appearance to the previous two figures. Mural thrombus is present behind the posterior leaflet of the mitral valve.

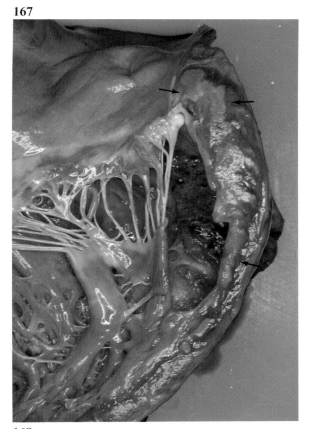

168 Myocardial infarct The appearance in a museum specimen of a transmural anterior infarct (1) with central necrosis and a surrounding haemorrhagic zone, for comparison with the three previous figures.

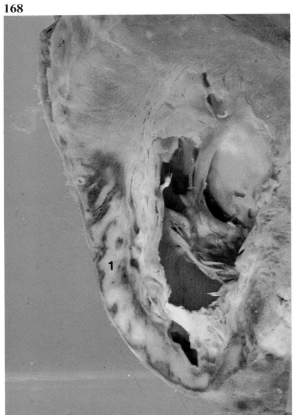

169 Myocardial infarct Healing of a myocardial infarct occurs by fibrous replacement of the damaged muscle and is complete after approximately six weeks. This transverse myocardial slice shows a fibrosing whole thickness infarct of the lateral wall of the left ventricle.

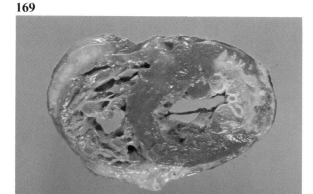

170 Myocardial infarct Endocardial fibrosis may result from organisation of mural thrombus as on the anterior wall and interventricular septum of this left ventricle opened down the lateral free border. Thinning of the wall in the septum and apex is also present.

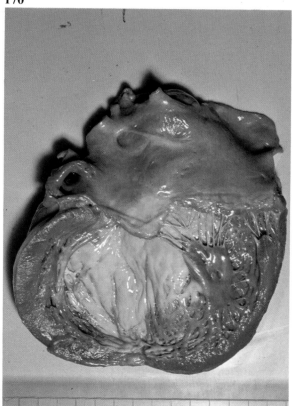

171 Myocardial infarct Following extensive loss of myocardium in a whole thickness infarct, thinning of the wall occurs as in this apical portion. In this heart the posterior wall of the right ventricle is involved as well as the left ventricle, due to a right coronary artery occlusion.

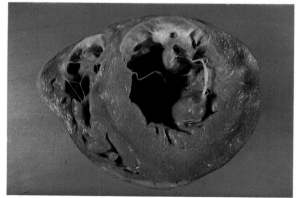

The following figures illustrate some of the microscopical appearances that are seen after the onset of myocardial ischaemia.

172 Myocardial infarction Oedema of muscle fibres may be seen with light microscopy approximately three to five hours after the onset of ischaemia. In this illustration all the myocardial fibres are oedematous being paler and wider than normal and with the cross-striations more spread out. (*H&E,* × 352)

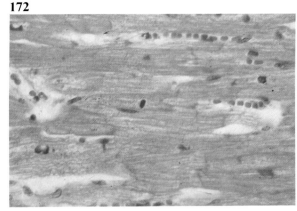

173 Myocardial infarction Before early muscle damage is discernible on an haematoxylin and eosin stain it may be detected by an haematoxylin basic fuchsin picric acid stain. Damaged fibres stain a brilliant red compared with the light brown colour of the normal fibres. In this figure striations are still visible in the damaged fibres. (× 352)

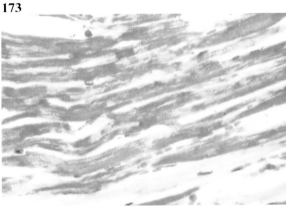

174 Myocardial infarction About six hours after infarction the muscle fibres stain more deeply with eosin and have a granular, banded cytoplasm, instead of the normal striations. Later the nuclei disappear. (*H&E,* × 352)

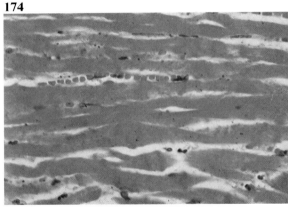

175 Myocardial infarction Early migration of polymorphonuclear leucocytes from a small vessel into the surrounding myocardium in a heart with a myocardial infarction of six hours' duration. This is usually the earliest time at which an acute inflammatory cell infiltrate becomes apparent in an area of infarction. (*H&E,* × 352)

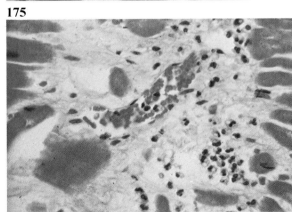

176 Myocardial infarction Polymorphonuclear leucocytes are now present amongst the necrotic myocardial fibres which have lost their nuclei and striations, and show increased staining with eosin compared with normal. The patient had a clinical history of myocardial ischaemia 24 hours before death. (*H&E*, × 352)

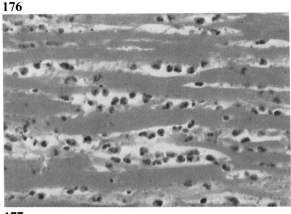

177 Myocardial infarction A dense polymorphonuclear leucocyte infiltrate may be present 48–60 hours after the onset of ischaemia with the necrosis of the muscle fibres becoming more obvious. (*H&E*, × 352)

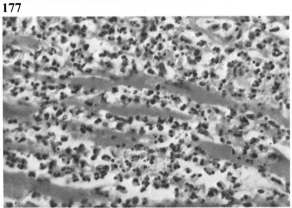

178 Myocardial infarction In a large infarct without any blood supply in the central zone the acute inflammatory infiltrate is confined to the edge, seen in the upper part of this illustration. (*H&E*, × 140)

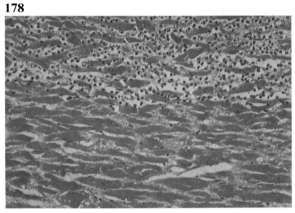

179 Myocardial infarction After a few days, in addition to necrosis of the muscle fibres, there is necrosis of inflammatory cells. (*H&E*, × 352)

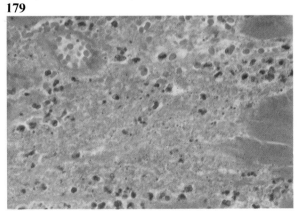

180 Myocardial infarction As the myocardial fibres are absorbed fibroblasts proliferate. This section is of the edge of an infarct with the viable muscle fibres on the right adjoining ischaemic vacuolated fibres, fibroblasts and mononuclear macrophages. (*H&E*, ×140)

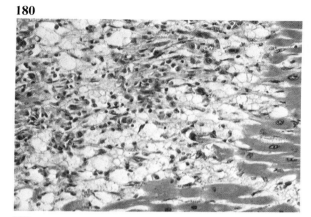

181 Myocardial infarction Collagen is gradually formed by the fibroblasts over the next few weeks. In this haematoxylin and eosin section the collagen stains a pale pink in contrast to the more red colour of the remaining muscle fibres. Moderately large thin walled blood vessels are present amongst the fibrous tissue. (*H&E*, ×88)

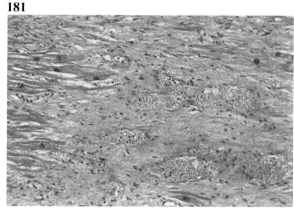

182 Myocardial infarction Collagenous tissue in a 'healing' infarct is more clearly delineated by the use of connective tissue stains such as the Martius scarlet blue staining method. (*MSB*, ×88)

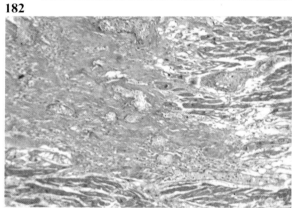

183 Myocardial infarction Following ischaemia in the subendocardial zone a few layers of muscle fibres often remain viable immediately underlying the endocardium (1) and also alongside the small arteries (*arrow*). The pale pink staining tissue is mature collagen. (*H&E*, ×22)

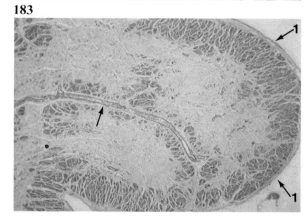

SOME COMPLICATIONS OF MYOCARDIAL INFARCTION

184 Ruptured ventricle A rupture in the lower third of the anterior wall of the left ventricle. This is the commonest site for a rupture which most often occurs during the first week after the onset of a transmural myocardial infarct.

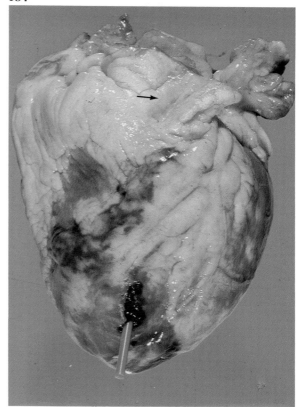

185 Mural thrombus A left ventricle opened to show recently formed mural thrombus attached to an area of infarction in the anterior apical region. Rupture of the wall has also occurred.

185

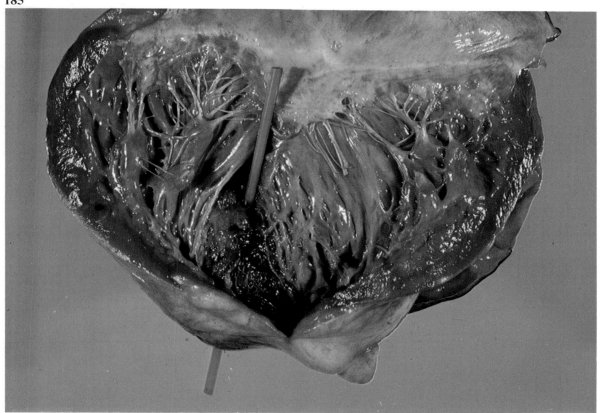

186 Mural thrombus In contrast to the previous figure, the mural thrombus (1) in this left ventricle is partially organised, with fibrous tissue already formed at the circumference.

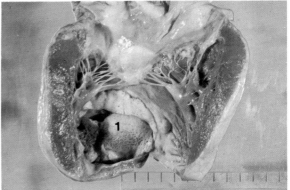

187 Ruptured interventricular septum A ragged perforation, indicated by a blue rod, in the lower part of an interventricular septum. This complication of myocardial infarction is uncommon. Initially the tear is often small and difficult to see but with healing tends to become a more clearly outlined hole (see **188**).

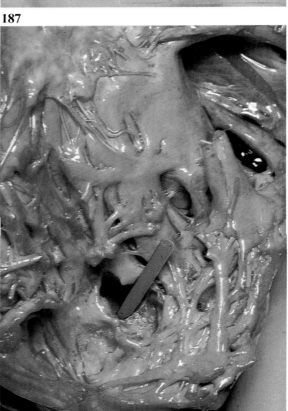

188 Ruptured interventricular septum View at operation for repair of a perforation (*arrow*) of an interventricular septum. It illustrates the optimum time to perform this operation when the surrounding infarcted muscle has been replaced by fibrous tissue.

    1 = ventricular wall
    2 = interventricular septum.

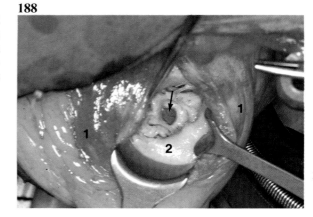

189 Papillary muscle infarction Papillary muscles in the left ventricle may fairly frequently be involved in myocardial infarction, as shown in this posterior papillary muscle (*arrow*).

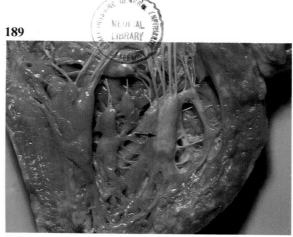

190 Ruptured papillary muscle A ruptured papillary muscle (*arrow*) of the left ventricle of the heart of a 53-year-old male who had had a myocardial infarction four days previously. Compared with the frequency of papillary infarction their rupture is uncommon.

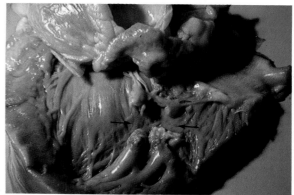

191 Papillary muscle fibrosis Close-up view of the cut upper ends of the papillary muscles (*arrowed*) of the left ventricle of a heart with a previous infarction of the posterior wall. The posterior papillary muscle, on the right, shows both endocardial and myocardial fibrosis.

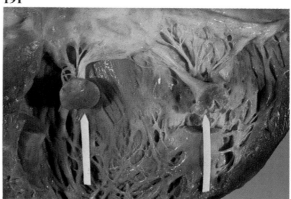

192 Papillary muscle fibrosis This excised valve viewed from below shows the upper part of a normal papillary muscle on the left and a fibrosed papillary muscle on the right (*arrow*). When extensive fibrous replacement of the myocardium of a papillary muscle occurs following ischaemia, mitral valve function may be affected with resulting regurgitation. If severe, valve replacement may be necessary.

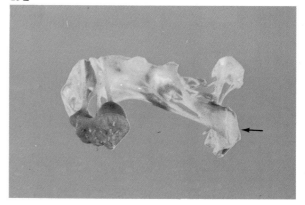

193 Ventricular aneurysm Aneurysms may develop following thinning and weakening of the infarcted myocardial wall. This figure illustrates a very large apical aneurysm of the left ventricle filled with laminated thrombus. The patient had a history of a myocardial infarction four years previously. (*Museum specimen*)

194 Ventricular aneurysm A left lateral view of a heart with an aneurysm of the posterior wall of the left ventricle. These are usually smaller and more basal in position compared with an anterior, apical, aneurysm. There was an old occlusion of the right coronary artery.

195 Ventricular aneurysm The aneurysm illustrated in the previous figure is here cut open to show thinning of the wall, mural thrombus and endocardial fibrosis.

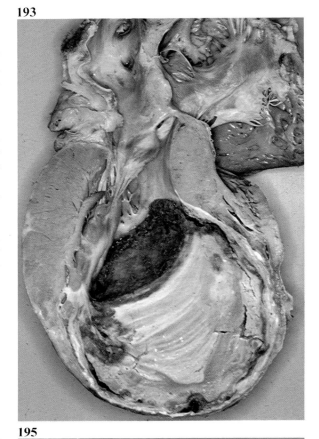

193

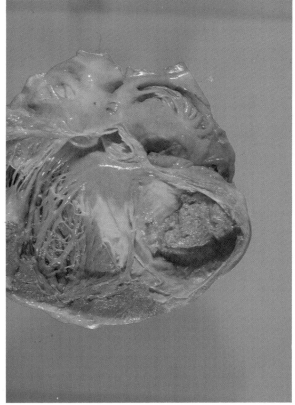

194

195

Myocardial vasculature following myocardial infarction

The x-rays in this section illustrate some of the abnormal vascular patterns that are seen in the myocardial wall following infarction.

196 & 197 Myocardial vascular pattern following myocardial infarction In hearts with considerable thinning and fibrosis of part of the ventricular wall, as illustrated in **196**, the x-ray of the thinned area shows loss of normal arterial pattern and only a few small supplying arteries remaining. (× 1.7, × 1.8)

196

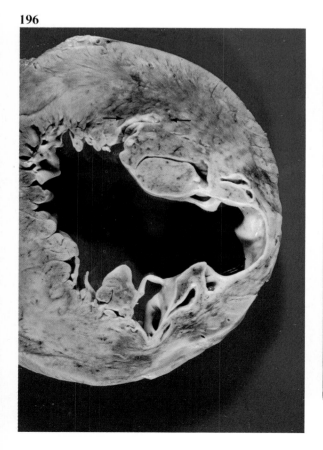

197

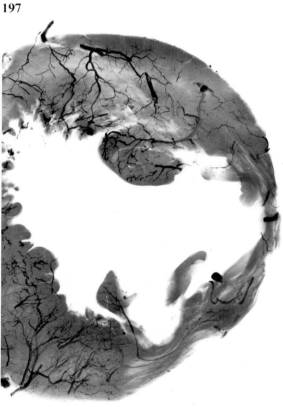

198 & 199 Myocardial vascular pattern following myocardial infarction In areas of infarction in which a moderate number of muscle fibres remain, collateral vessels may be formed in the 'scarred' area. Figure **198** illustrates the gross appearance of such an area in the postero-lateral wall (*arrow*) of a 5mm ventricular slice, while **199**, an x-ray, illustrates collateral arteries coursing circumferentially (*arrow*) in the middle of this part of the wall. (×2.25)

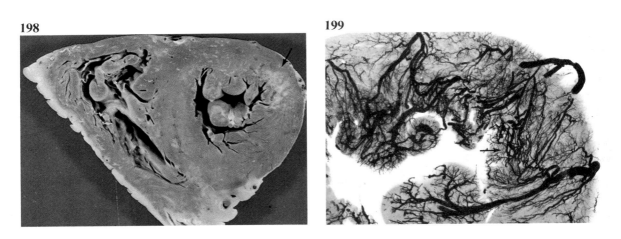

200 Myocardial vascular pattern following myocardial infarction An abnormal extensive plexus of vessels may form, in the inner half of the left ventricular wall in areas of myocardial ischaemia in hearts with severe atheroma of all the main coronary arteries. In this microradiograph of a 5mm midventricular slice the plexus is present in the posterior, lateral and majority of the anterior wall of the left ventricle. This type of vascular pattern characteristically occurs in a 'laminar' type of myocardial infarction (see **158**). (×1.8)

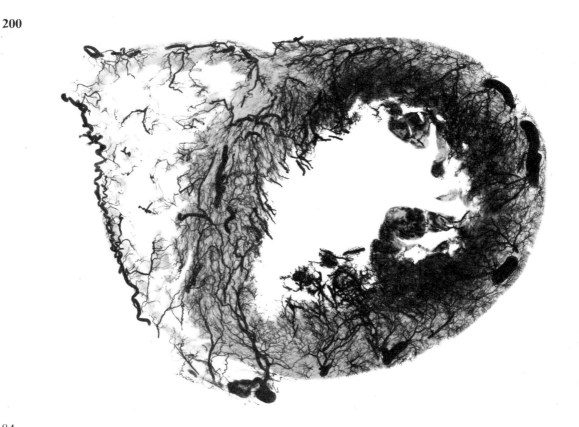

201 Myocardial vascular pattern following myocardial infarction High magnification of an x-ray of a 2.5mm slice of the lateral wall of a left ventricle, shows that the plexus illustrated in the previous figure is composed of both radially and circumferentially running vessels. The vascular pattern in the outer half of the wall on the right of the figure is normal. (× 6)

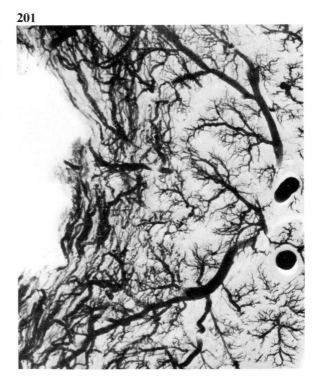

202 Myocardial vascular pattern following myocardial infarction Development of a functioning collateral system may not be extensive in patients with coronary artery disease affecting mainly one coronary artery. This microradiograph of a midventricular slice from a heart with an occlusion of the left main trunk shows filling by radio-opaque medium mainly confined to the right coronary tree. This heart was from a patient who died three hours after the initial symptoms of myocardial ischaemia. (× 0.75)

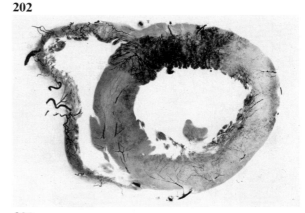

203 Myocardial venous pattern following myocardial infarction In areas of fibrosis, resulting from coronary artery disease, there is loss of normal venous pattern (see **111** and **112**) and interruption of main drainage veins. (× 4)

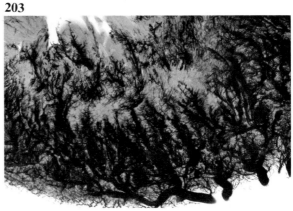

204 Myocardial venous pattern following myocardial infarction In hearts with generalised severe coronary artery disease a 'plexus' of veins may be present in the inner half to two-thirds of the wall, with loss of the normal large drainage veins. This may result in stasis of the blood in this area. This 'plexus' is the venous component corresponding to the arterial 'plexus' of vessels shown in **200** and **201**. (× 3)

205 Myocardial venous pattern following myocardial infarction A higher power of the plexus of veins, illustrated in the previous figure, shows the majority of vessels coursing circumferentially with absence of normal drainage veins. (× 16)

204

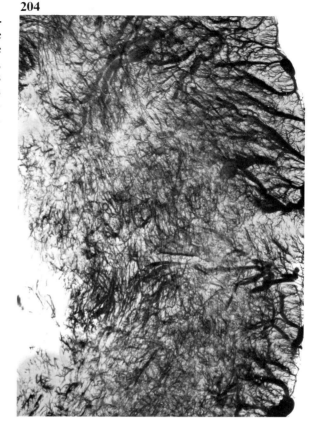

205

206

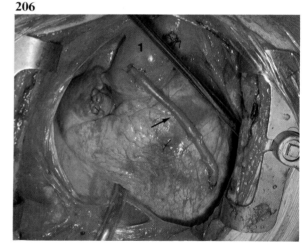

206 Saphenous vein bypass graft An important surgical treatment for coronary artery disease is the use of a saphenous vein bypass graft. This figure is an operative view of the insertion of one of these grafts (*arrow*) to bypass a localised area of severe atheroma in the left anterior descending coronary artery. The upper end of the vein graft is anastomosed to the aorta a few centimetres above the aortic valve.

1 = aorta

207 Saphenous vein bypass graft A saphenous vein bypass graft (*arrow*) that was inserted 15 months previously into the lower end of the anterior descending coronary artery. The lumen of the vein was still patent.

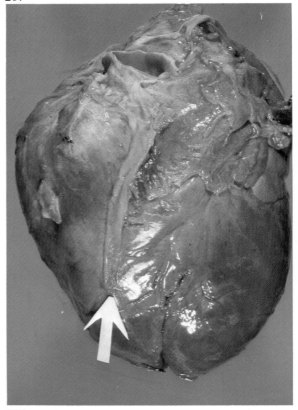

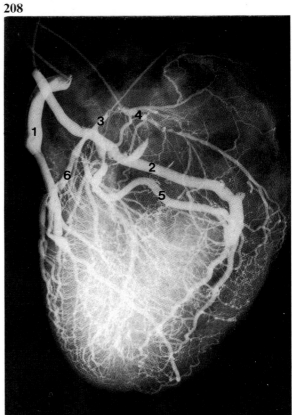

208 Saphenous vein bypass graft An oblique lateral whole heart x-ray to demonstrate filling of the entire coronary artery tree following injection of radio-opaque medium down two saphenous vein bypass grafts. One vein graft is inserted into the distal part of the anterior descending coronary artery. The second vein graft is inserted into the distal part of the left circumflex coronary artery. The right coronary artery is a very small vessel.

    1 = vein graft anterior descending artery
    2 = vein graft left circumflex artery
    3 = left coronary artery
    4 = right coronary artery
    5 = left circumflex artery
    6 = left anterior descending artery

Hypertrophy of the ventricles

Hypertrophy of the myocardial fibres results in an increase in heart size and weight. It may occur as a physiological response to sustained physical exercise, but more commonly it is the result of pathological conditions such as hypertension, heart valve disease and lung disease.

209–212 Hypertrophy These four figures are all anterior views of unopened hearts illustrating the appearance of:
- **209** A normal heart.
- **210** A heart with considerable left ventricular hypertrophy.
- **211** A heart with considerable right ventricular hypertrophy.
- **212** A heart with both right and left ventricular hypertrophy.

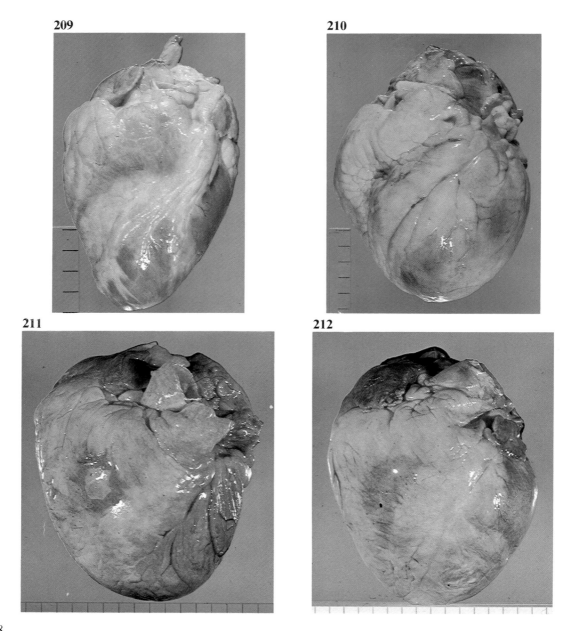

213–215 Hypertrophy The most effective macroscopic method of assessing the myocardial wall thickness in relation to the size of the ventricular chamber is to study transverse ventricular slices. The following three figures are of transverse mid-ventricular slices illustrating:

213 A heart with concentric left ventricular hypertrophy due to benign hypertension.

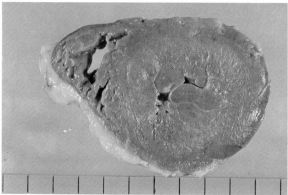

214 A heart with right ventricular hypertrophy and dilatation (cor pulmonale) due to chronic obstructive airways disease.

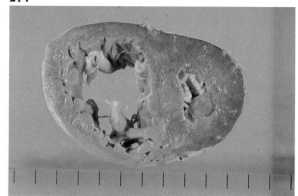

215 A heart with left and right ventricular dilatation and hypertrophy due to mitral valve disease with resulting pulmonary hypertension.

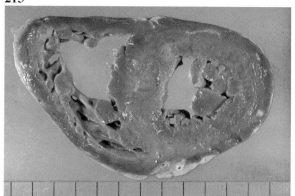

216 Hypertrophy An opened left ventricle with considerable hypertrophy of the myocardium due to benign hypertension. Note the thickened papillary muscles. For accurate assessment of the degree of hypertrophy, weighing of the excised left ventricle and interventricular septum is necessary. It is important that all epicardial fat is carefully removed before dissection.

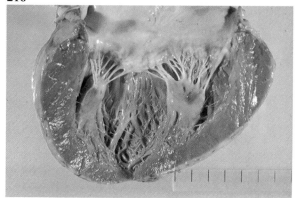

217 Hypertrophy An opened right ventricle with hypertrophy of the myocardium, occurring in a patient with cor pulmonale. As with the left ventricle, the variation in dilatation of the cavity makes measurement of wall thickness an inaccurate method of estimating hypertrophy and weighing of the excised free wall should be carried out.

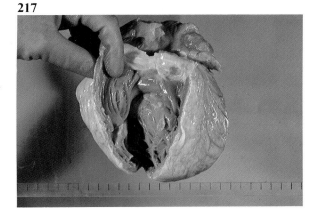

218 Acromegaly Massive cardiomegaly in a 39-year-old man with acromegaly who died of congestive cardiac failure. The heart weighed 1240g and showed enlargement of all chambers with hypertrophy of the muscle. For comparison, on the right, is a normal 380g museum specimen heart.

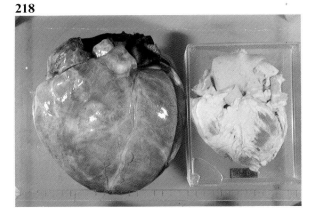

219 & 220 Hypertrophy Normal (**219**) and hypertrophied (**220**) left ventricular myocardial fibres photographed at the same magnification. Note the difference in muscle fibre thickness and size and shape of the nuclei. (× 550)

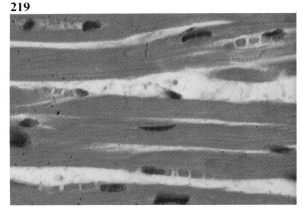

Primary cardiomyopathies

The term 'primary cardiomyopathy' is commonly used to describe cardiac diseases of unknown cause primarily involving heart muscle. Known causes, such as valve disease, hypertension, coronary artery disease and congenital abnormalities must be excluded before the diagnosis of a primary cardiomyopathy can be considered.

Three main clinical categories are usually described:

(1) Congestive cardiomyopathy characterised by poor systolic function with failure to empty adequately. (See 221–223)

(2) Hypertrophic cardiomyopathy characterised by impaired diastolic compliance which leads to resistance to ventricular filling in diastole. There may or may not be an obstructive element. (See 224–229)

(3) Obliterative cardiomyopathy characterised by obliteration of the ventricular cavities. (See 230–236)

A fourth type, restrictive cardiomyopathy, when the ventricular wall is affected by such conditions as amyloid, is sometimes described as a primary type of cardiomyopathy but it is rare.

221 Primary cardiomyopathy, congestive type An example of the characteristic globe shaped, dilated, left ventricle of an enlarged heart with congestive cardiomyopathy. Myocardial hypertrophy is present, but is not obvious due to marked dilatation of the cavity. The papillary muscles in this condition appear normal or flat and shrunken. The other chambers of the heart were also dilated.

221

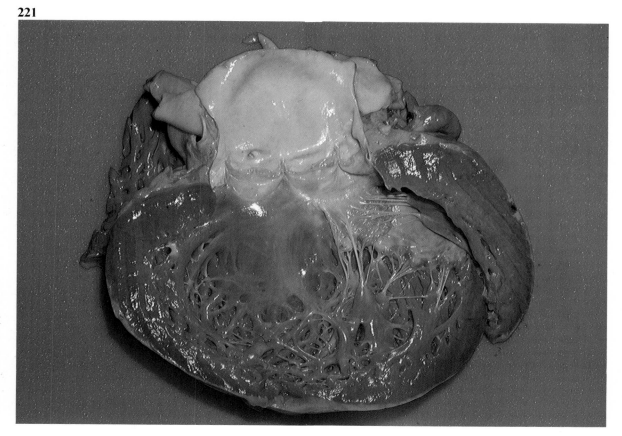

222 Primary cardiomyopathy, congestive type
Hearts with congestive cardiomyopathy may have
scattered endocardial thrombi in the left ventricle,
particularly in the interstices of the muscle columns.
The appearance and distribution of these thrombi
differ from those seen in endomyocardial fibrosis
(see **231**).

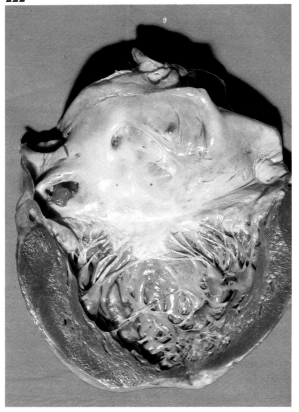

223 Primary cardiomyopathy, congestive type The
myocardium of a heart with congestive cardiomyopathy showing long runs of attenuated,
degenerate muscle fibres with some nuclei large and
hyperchromatic. Occasional fibres are hypertrophic. Mild vacuolation of the centre of some
degenerate fibres is present while there is also
increased fibrosis and scattered inflammatory cells.
(× 140)

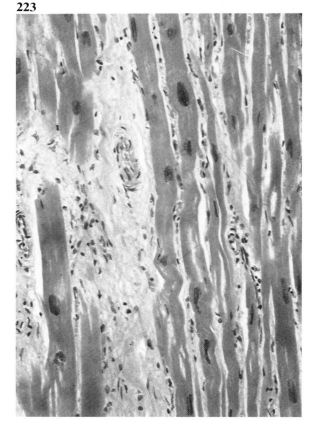

224 Primary cardiomyopathy, hypertrophic type
Lateral view of a sagittal section of the anterior wall
of the left ventricle and the interventricular septum.
The latter shows disproportionate hypertrophy
compared with the remainder of the wall and is
bulging and obstructing the aortic outflow tract
(*arrow*). Note the characteristic small left
ventricular cavity. This is the classical asymmetrical
type of hypertrophic cardiomyopathy. White radio-
opaque medium is present in the coronary arteries.
(*Museum specimen*)

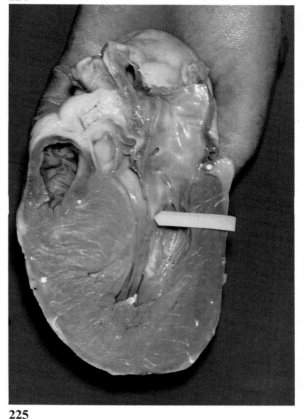
224

**225 & 226 Primary cardiomyopathy, hypertrophic
type** The ventricular hypertrophy in hypertrophic
cardiomyopathy is not always localised to the
interventricular septum, and some hearts show
symmetrical hypertrophy of the whole left ventricle.
These illustrations compare transverse ventricular
slices from (**225**) a heart with concentric, hypertrophic cardiomyopathy involving the free wall and
interventricular septum equally and (**226**) an
asymmetrical type with the interventricular septum
showing disproportionate hypertrophy compared
with the free left ventricular wall.

225

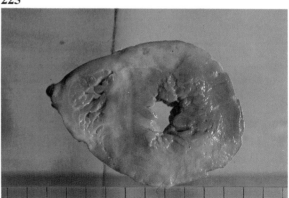
226

227 Primary cardiomyopathy, hypertrophic type An opened left ventricle of an enlarged heart with diffuse concentric, hypertrophic cardiomyopathy, showing an area of endocardial fibrosis (*arrow*) beneath the aortic valve. This fibrosis is caused by the anterior cusp of the mitral valve hitting against the bulging interventricular septum. This feature, when present, is diagnostic of hypertrophic obstructive cardiomyopathy. In this heart, the appearance of the cavity is not typical as it is dilated because the patient developed cardiac failure.

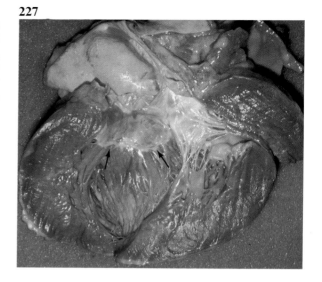

228 Primary cardiomyopathy, hypertrophic type Myocardium of a heart with this condition showing disordered interlacing hypertrophic fibres, but with some variability in size of the fibres. Another characteristic is that the fibres show a swirling or whorled pattern. Interstitial and focal areas of fibrosis may also be present. (*H&E,* × 140)

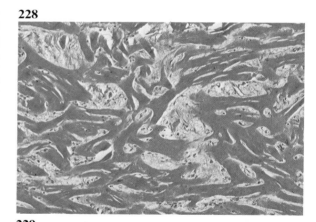

229 Primary cardiomyopathy, hypertrophic type Close-up of short hypertrophic interlacing fibres with bizarre, prominent nuclei. (*H&E,* × 352)

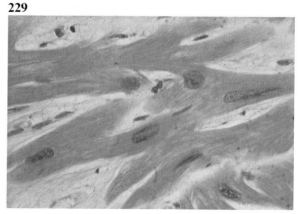

230 Primary cardiomyopathy, obliterative type, endomyocardial fibrosis Characteristic notching of the apex of the right ventricle (*arrow*) in endomyocardial fibrosis. This is due to the fibrous obliteration of the cavity of this ventricle. This disease of unknown aetiology may affect either the right or left ventricle, or both.

230

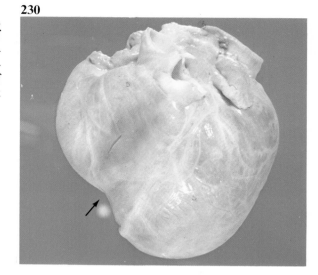

231 Primary cardiomyopathy, obliterative type, endomyocardial fibrosis Endocardial thrombus involving mainly the apex of the left ventricle in a heart with an early stage endomyocardial fibrosis. The thrombus gradually becomes organised into fibrous tissue as illustrated in the next two figures, which also show other characteristic areas of involvement of the left ventricle in EMF.

231

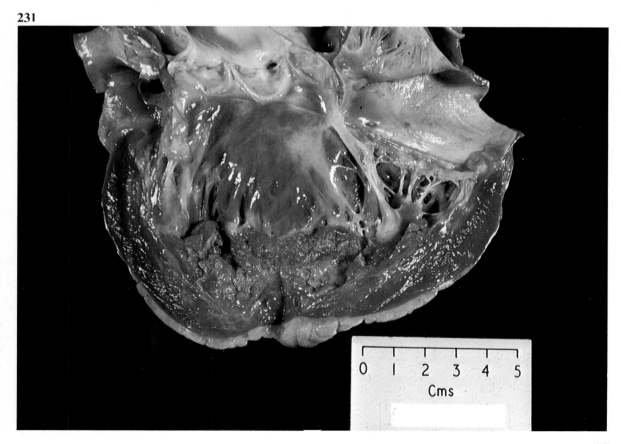

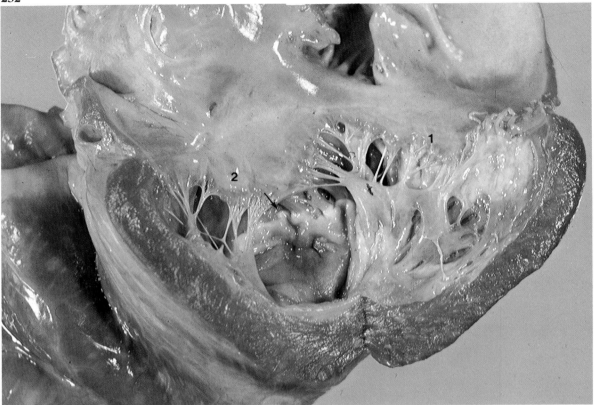

232 Primary cardiomyopathy, obliterative type, endomyocardial fibrosis A later stage of the disease in the left ventricle compared to the previous figure. Extensive fibrosis involves the apex and the wall adjacent to the posterior cusps (1) of the mitral valve. This part of the valve becomes secondarily bound down to the thrombus and fibrous tissue with resulting incompetence. Beneath the unaffected anterior cusp (2) of the mitral valve a ridge of endocardial fibrous tissue (*arrow*) is seen at the commencement of the outflow tract. One of the reasons for the characteristic distribution of the endocardial lesions is the low shear force of the affected areas associated with the blood flow pattern within the left ventricle.

233 Primary cardiomyopathy, obliterative type, endomyocardial fibrosis A late stage of the disease with the endocardial fibrosis involving all the left ventricle except the outflow tract. Note the fibrous tissue surrounding and binding down the posterior papillary muscles (*arrow*). Valve involvement is usually confined to the mitral and tricuspid with the pulmonary valve only rarely affected.

233

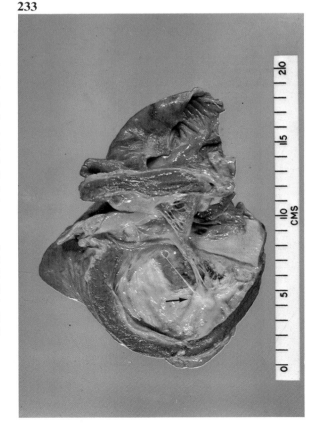

234 & 235 Primary cardiomyopathy, obliterative type, endomyocardial fibrosis The extent to which the ventricular cavity may become obliterated is shown in these two transverse ventricular slices of hearts injected with yellow and blue radio-opaque media respectively. The cavity of the right ventricle of the first heart, with relatively early stage disease, is obliterated by organising thrombus (1) and in the second heart, with late stage disease, by fibrous tissue (2). In contrast to the hearts in the previous three figures the right ventricle is affected more severely than the left.

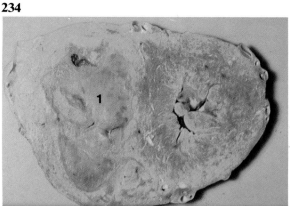

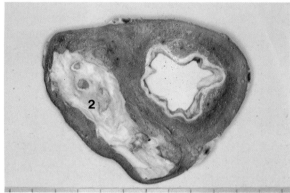

236 Primary cardiomyopathy, obliterative type, endomyocardial fibrosis Myocardial fibrosis, mainly subendocardial in distribution (1), is seen in this disease in addition to the endocardial fibrosis (2). The small myocardial blood vessels appear normal. (*VG*, ×18)

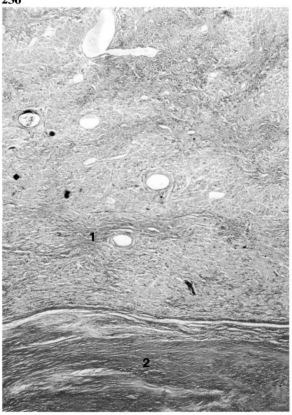

237 Isolated endocardial fibroelastosis This disease of unknown aetiology is often considered, for convenience, with the primary cardiomyopathies of the obliterative type, although basically it is a disease of endocardium. It is usually seen in infants and young children and although chambers of both sides of the heart may be affected the left side is more commonly involved. The illustrated heart is from a 3-day-old infant and shows a small hypertrophied left ventricle with a small cavity lined by a smooth, white, markedly thickened endocardium.

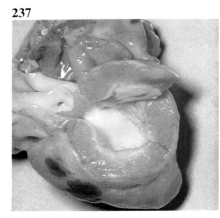

238 Isolated endocardial fibroelastosis The considerable thickening of the endocardium in this condition is well illustrated where the inner wall of the left ventricle has been cut. This heart is from a child who died aged 16 months, and the cavity is dilated compared with the heart in the previous figure.

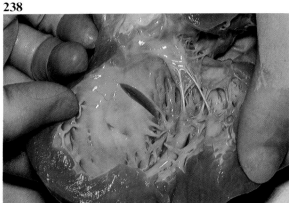

239 Isolated endocardial fibroelastosis Thickened fibrotic endocardium as seen in a haematoxylin and eosin stained section. (× 140)

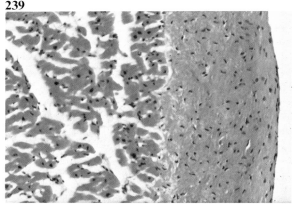

240 Isolated endocardial fibroelastosis An elastic van Gieson stain showing the elastic and collagen fibres in the thickened endocardium. Collagen, red. Elastic = black. Myocardium = brown. (*EVG*, ×352)

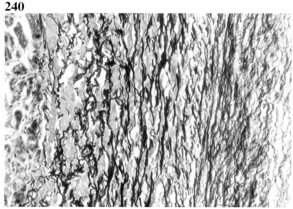

Rheumatic heart disease

Rheumatic heart disease occurs as part of a systemic disease of connective tissue resulting from an abnormal immune response to a previous Group A, ß haemolytic, streptococcal infection. Nowadays in many countries death is uncommon in acute rheumatic carditis and the importance of heart involvement lies mainly in the continuing damage of the valves, particularly the mitral and aortic, in chronic rheumatic heart disease.

241 & 242 Rheumatic heart disease Aschoff's nodes are the characteristic and pathognomonic granulomatous lesion of rheumatic heart disease. These nodes are seen approximately one month after the onset of the disease and may be found in any, or all, of the three layers of the heart. Figure **241** shows them present in stromal connective tissue of the myocardium which is usually most abundant around blood vessels. Figure **242** illustrates a fully developed Aschoff's node with central fibrinoid material surrounded by histiocytes and scanty lymphocytes, plasma and giant cells. The characteristic histiocytic, or Anitschkow, cells, are large with a slightly basophilic cytoplasm. Their nuclei contain a central bar of chromatin from which fine strands radiate outwards. When cut in cross-section the nuclei may resemble 'owls' eyes' and in longitudinal section 'caterpillars'. The giant, or Aschoff cells, typically contain 3–4 centrally placed nuclei and are also of histiocytic origin. (*H&E*, ×88, ×220)

241

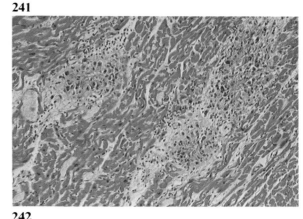

242

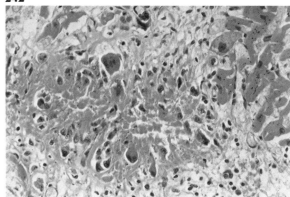

243 Rheumatic heart disease, Aschoff's nodes The appearance of these nodes varies in the different stages of evolution and involution. One of the named varieties is the fibrillary type, here situated alongside a blood vessel with myocardium on the right. The histiocytic cells are elongated and spindle shaped and mainly orientated in a longitudinal axis. (*H&E*, × 352)

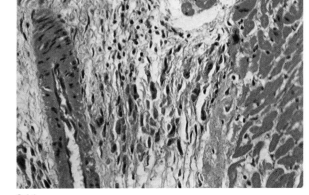

244 Rheumatic heart disease, Aschoff's node A small node (*arrow*) present in the endocardium of an atrial appendage biopsy taken during surgical replacement of a mitral valve. It is interesting that these lesions may be found as much as 20–30 years after the initial rheumatic fever, but do not appear to affect the post-operative course of the patient. (*H&E*, × 88)

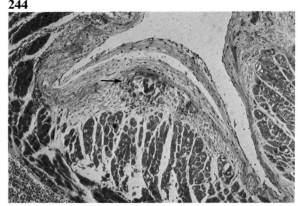

245 Rheumatic heart disease, arteritis An arteritis may be present, as shown here by the presence of an Aschoff's node (*arrow*) in the wall of a small coronary blood vessel. (*H&E*, × 140)

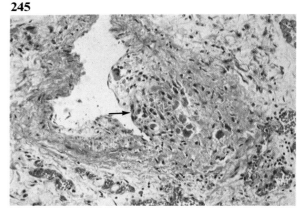

246 Acute rheumatic heart disease Acute rheumatic endocarditis with small translucent nodules along the contact edge of a slightly thickened mitral valve. Similar lesions are present on the aortic valve seen on the left. This heart, from a 15-year-old boy, was enlarged, with the left ventricular cavity dilated and globe shaped and with thickening of its wall. (*Museum specimen*)

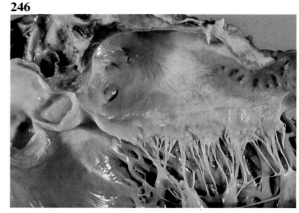

247 Acute rheumatic heart disease Close-up view of the nodules of acute rheumatic endocarditis on the mitral valve illustrated in the previous figure. (*Museum specimen*)

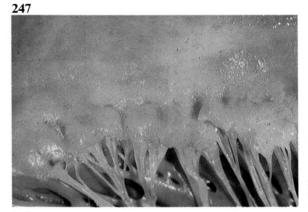

248 Acute rheumatic heart disease This heart with acute rheumatic heart disease shows nodules present not only along the contact margin of the mitral valve, but also on the chordae tendineae and mural endocardium (*arrow*). (*Museum specimen*)

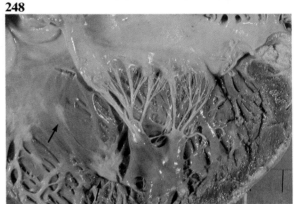

249 Acute rheumatic heart disease An acute mitral valve lesion with fibrinoid degeneration within the valve margin merging with an overlying fibrinoid vegetation. Aschoff's nodes may also develop in the valve but are not illustrated. (*H&E,* × 88)

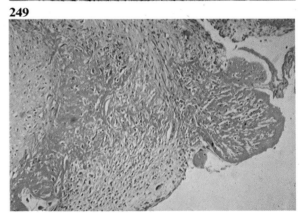

250 Rheumatic heart disease, mitral valve In chronic rheumatic heart disease the most serious changes are in the valves. This close-up shows the late stages of the disease in a mitral valve, which is the most commonly affected valve, either alone or in combination with the aortic valve. In addition to the fibrous thickening of the valve leaflets and adhesions of the commissures the chordae tendineae are characteristically thickened and shortened. In addition, on the upper surface of this valve small vegetations are present.

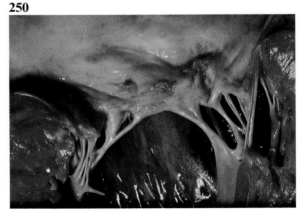

251

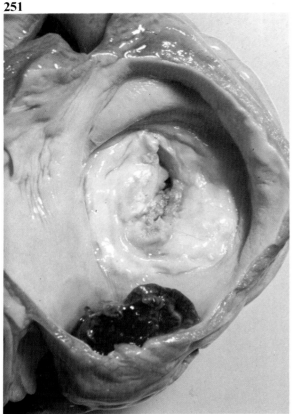

252

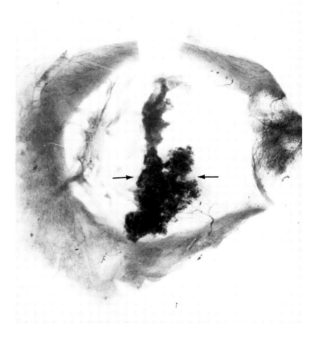

251 Rheumatic heart disease, mitral valve The atrium has been cut away to show a grossly stenotic, calcified, mitral valve resulting from rheumatic heart disease. Only a slit-like opening remains. Ante-mortem thrombus is present in the left auricular appendage.

252 Rheumatic heart disease, mitral valve This x-ray shows more clearly than can be appreciated by naked eye the extent of calcification (*arrow*) that is present in the severely diseased mitral valve in the previous figure. The less dense black tissue at the circumference is the myocardium at the valve ring containing small arteries filled by radio-opaque injection medium. (× 2)

253 Rheumatic heart disease, mitral valve Section of a mitral valve with gross calcification (*arrow*) following chronic rheumatic heart disease. It also illustrates dense fibrous thickening of the valve and increased vascularity, indicated by black-staining radio-opaque medium within the blood vessels. Chronic inflammatory cells were present focally in this valve. (*H&E*, × 8.8)

253

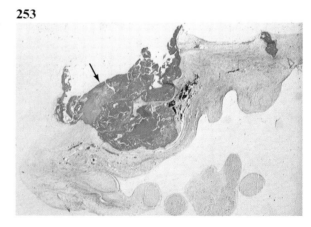

254 Rheumatic heart disease, aortic valve An aortic valve with mild thickening of the cusps and the beginning of commissural adhesions (*arrow*) resulting from rheumatic heart disease.

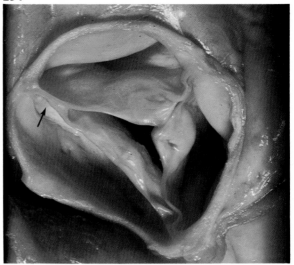

255 Rheumatic heart disease, aortic valve An opened aortic valve with more extensive commissural adhesions (*arrow*) and valve cusp thickening compared with the previous figure. Calcification is also present.

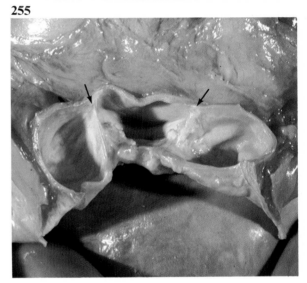

256 Rheumatic heart disease, aortic valve A stenotic and incompetent aortic valve severely affected by rheumatic heart disease. Fusion of all three commissures has resulted in a small central triangular orifice. The appearances of this valve should be compared with the two other main forms of isolated aortic stenosis in adults, illustrated in **290** and **291**.

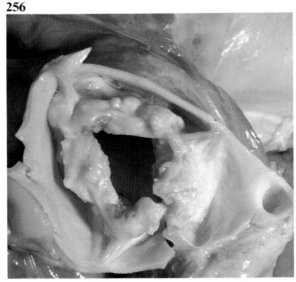

257 Rheumatic heart disease, tricuspid valve An opened tricuspid valve with a characteristic thick crescent shaped valve leaflet due to rheumatic heart disease. In addition to the fusion of the thickened cusps there is also thickening of the chordae tendineae, but this is not illustrated. The gross changes in a tricuspid valve are never as severe as those seen in mitral and aortic valves and calcification is rare. The tricuspid valve is usually only affected when both the mitral and aortic valves are diseased while less commonly all four heart valves are involved. The incidence of valve involvement is related to the height of the closing pressures at the valve, which is approximately systolic blood pressure for the mitral, diastolic for the aortic and the pulmonary pressure for the tricuspid and pulmonary valves.

258 Rheumatic heart disease, hypertrophy Left ventricular hypertrophy resulting from rheumatic aortic and mitral valve disease. The thickening of the mitral valve is clearly seen, but the aortic valve is not visible.

259 Rheumatic heart disease, atrial dilatation Gross dilatation of the left atrium occurring in a heart with rheumatic mitral valve disease. Note that the openings of the four pulmonary veins, filled with post-mortem clot, are widely separated. This dilation nearly always results from mitral incompetence, with or without stenosis, and is most commonly seen in rheumatic heart disease.

257

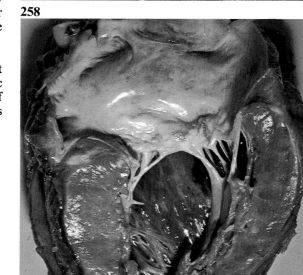

258

259

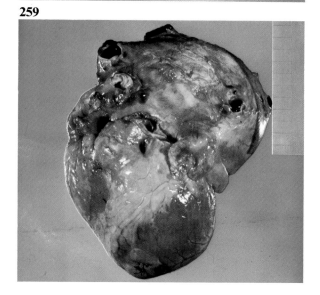

260 Rheumatic heart disease, post operative A severely diseased mitral valve with two splits (*arrow*) produced by a previous valvotomy. The patient died subsequently of cardiac failure.

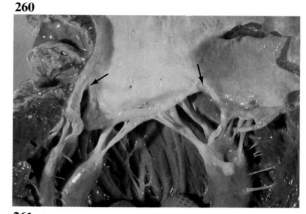

261 Rheumatic heart disease, post operative An excised mitral valve and chordae tendineae severely affected by rheumatic heart disease removed to allow insertion of an artificial valve.

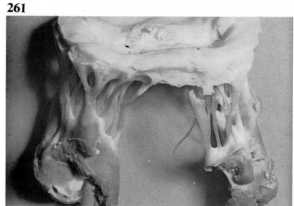

262 Rheumatic heart disease, post operative Superior view of a recently inserted artificial Starr-Edwards ball valve replacing a diseased mitral valve.

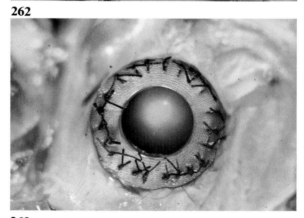

263 Rheumatic heart disease. Post operative complication—infective endocarditis Infective vegetations (*arrow*) adherent to the upper edge of a Starr-Edwards ball valve replacing an aortic valve.

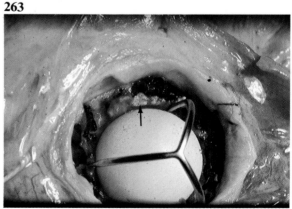

264 Rheumatic heart disease. Post operative complication—focal necrosis In this transverse ventricular slice focal, and mainly subendocardial, areas of ischaemic necrosis (*arrow*) are present in the posterior half of the interventricular septum, and posterior wall of the left ventricle. They occurred following an operation for a mitral valve replacement for rheumatic heart disease in a patient with no significant coronary artery atheroma. This type of necrosis is not specific to patients with rheumatic heart disease and may follow any cardiac surgery.

265 Rheumatic heart disease. Post operative complication—endocardial fibrosis Ventricular endocardial fibrosis may develop following insertion of artificial valves. The distribution of the fibrosis is primarily determined by mechanical factors and an altered flow pattern of blood within the left ventricle.

266 Rheumatic heart disease. Post operative complication—endocardial fibrosis The thickness of the ventricular endocardial fibrosis of the heart in the previous figure is more clearly seen following formalin fixation. The ball valve replacing the mitral valve is viewed from below.

267 Rheumatic heart disease. Post operative complication—endocardial fibrosis The thickened endocardium illustrated in the previous two figures is composed of fibrous and elastic tissue. Fibrous tissue = red. Myocardium = brown. Elastic tissue = black. (*EVG*, ×22)

264
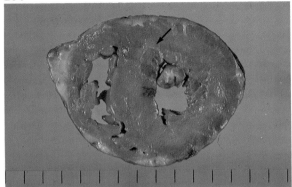

265
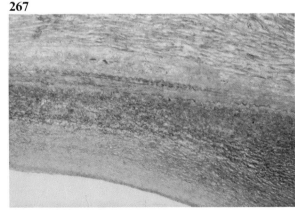

266
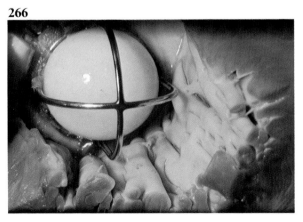

267

Other connective tissue disorders

Important connective tissue disorders, other than rheumatic fever, are illustrated in this section. Namely: rheumatoid arthritis, systemic lupus erythematosus, scleroderma and polyarteritis nodosa.

268 Rheumatoid heart disease In rheumatoid arthritis the heart may uncommonly be involved but only in patients with severe joint disease. This posterior view shows pale rheumatoid nodules scattered within the myocardium. Foci of haemorrhage are also present. The appearances of the interior of this heart are illustrated in the next two figures.

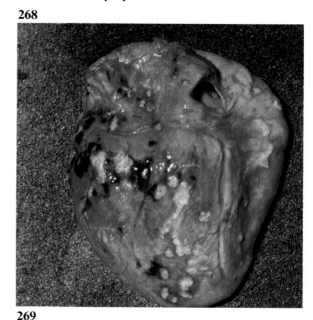

269 Rheumatoid heart disease The opened left ventricle showing rheumatoid nodules scattered in the myocardium, papillary muscles and mitral valve.

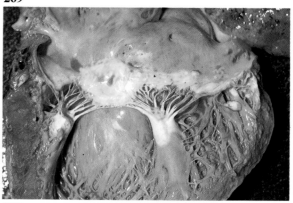

270 Rheumatoid heart disease The left outflow tract with coalescing rheumatoid nodules extending up to the aortic valve. The cusps (*arrow*) of the valve show no commissural adhesion but are contracted and thickened due to a rheumatoid valvulitis. Disease of the aortic valve is more commonly associated with a rheumatoid aortitis rather than with a generalised cardiac involvement.

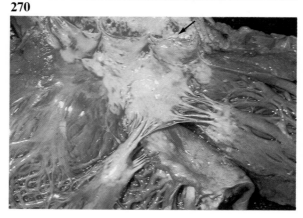

271 Rheumatoid disease Microscopical appearance of a mitral valve severely affected by rheumatoid disease and showing extensive granulomatous formation. A deep red staining area of fibrinoid necrosis (*arrow*) is surrounded by a blue staining cellular infiltrate of mononuclear cells. The pale pink staining tissue is fibrous tissue. Non-specific inflammation of valves may also occur in rheumatoid cardiac or aortic disease. (*H&E*, × 55)

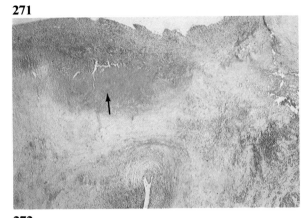

272 Systemic lupus erythematosus In this connective tissue disorder the valves of the heart may show characteristic lesions. The mitral is the most frequently affected valve followed by the aortic with the tricuspid and pulmonary less commonly involved. Illustrated here are red flat spreading lesions of atypical verrucous endocarditis of SLE, also referred to as Libman-Sacks endocarditis. The appearance of these vegetations varies and they may be more yellowish and nodular and extend onto the atrial and ventricular myocardium. Pericarditis and myocardial and coronary artery lesions may also be present.

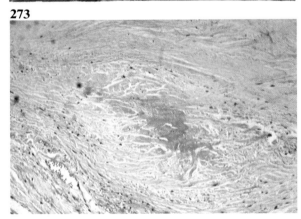

273 Systemic lupus erythematosus The histology of SLE is characterised by deeply eosinophilic areas of fibrinoid degeneration associated with a minimal mononuclear infiltrate and some fibroblastic proliferation. This illustration shows fibrinoid degeneration at the edge of a mitral valve. (× 220)

274 Scleroderma In this connective tissue disease there may be widespread myocardial degeneration with fibrous tissue replacement as illustrated in the thinned papillary muscles and free wall of this opened left ventricle. The heart was from a 53-year-old female.

274

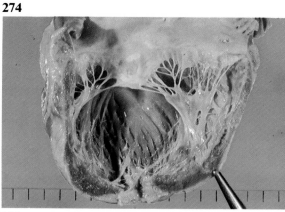

275

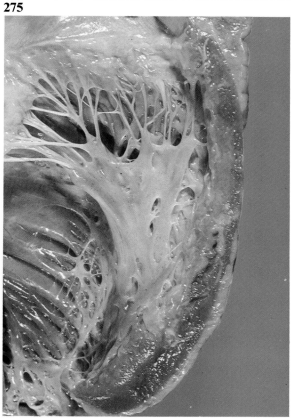

275 Scleroderma Higher magnification of the thinned lateral wall and posterior papillary muscle of the left ventricle of the heart illustrated in the previous figure. Pale pinkish-white fibrous tissue is extensively replacing the red myocardium.

276

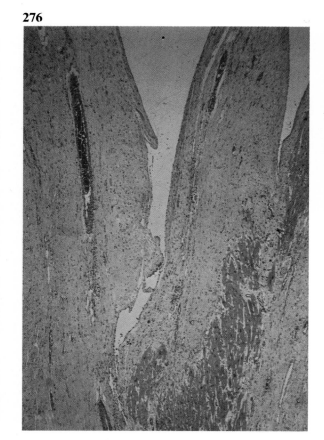

276 Scleroderma Extensive, focal, fibrous replacement of muscle fibres in the subendocardium and columnae carneae of the heart illustrated in the previous two figures. (*H&E, ×44*)

277–280 Polyarteritis nodosa In this disease, which is considered to be a connective tissue disorder, the coronary arteries are commonly affected. Macroscopic evidence of vessel involvement may be apparent when weakness of the wall of the extramyocardial portion of the arteries results in microaneurysm formation. Figure **277** shows multiple aneurysms along the coronary arteries of the heart of a young adult male who died of systemic polyarteritis nodosa. (*Museum specimen*)

Figures **278–280** illustrate some of the microscopical appearances that may be seen in this disease. The first two arteries are intramyocardial and the third extramyocardial.

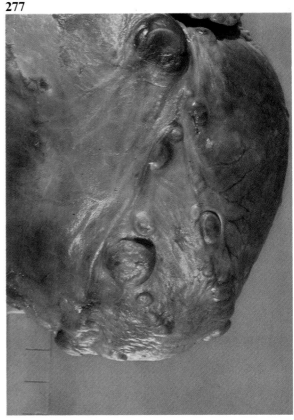

Figure **278** shows fibrinoid necrosis in the inner part of the wall associated with loss of normal architecture, but only a scanty inflammatory cell infiltrate is present in the wall.

Figure **279** shows a more severely affected artery with considerable inflammation of the wall.

The artery in **280** shows a late stage of the vessel disease with marked intimal fibrosis and almost complete obliteration of the lumen. (*H&E,* × 140, × 140, × 55)

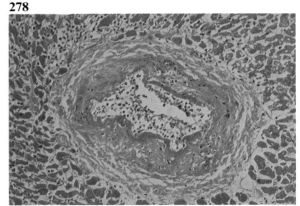

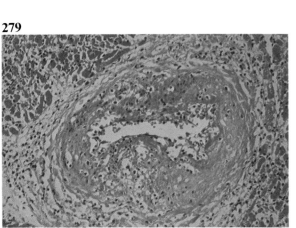

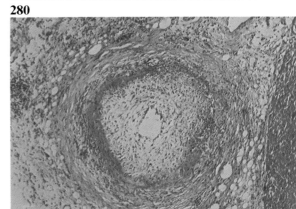

Syphilis

The heart and aorta may be affected in syphilis, although this type of involvement is now uncommon in many countries. The most serious lesion is an aortitis occurring in the tertiary stage with the resulting destruction and dilatation of the wall, causing stretch lesions of the aortic valve. Myocardial involvement by a localised gumma in the tertiary stage or interstitial myocarditis occurring in congenital syphilis are rarely seen.

281 Syphilis, aortic aneurysm An aneurysm of the ascending aorta (*arrow*) resulting from a weakening of the wall by a syphilitic mesoaortitis occurring in the tertiary stage of the disease.

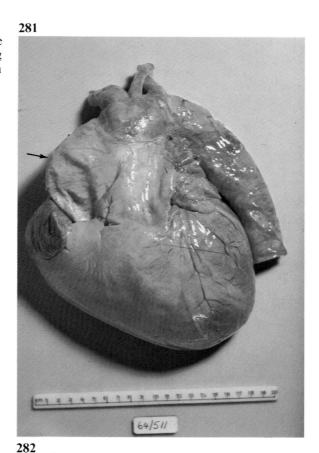

282 Syphilis, aortic aneurysm The same heart as illustrated in the previous figure opened to show the aortic aneurysm, an incompetent aortic valve and resulting hypertrophied left ventricle. The scarred appearance of the intimal surface of this aorta is due to atheroma superimposed on a syphilitic meso-aortitis.

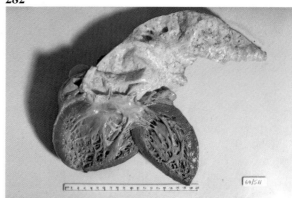

283 Syphilis, aortic valve A close-up view of an opened incompetent syphilitic aortic valve. There is obvious widening of the commissures with the cusps having rolled, thickened upper edges. The latter are stretch lesions and the result of damage produced by regurgitant blood stream. Microscopy shows this free margin thickening to be composed of dense collagen. This type of stretch lesion is not specific to syphilis and may also occur in other diseases such as ankylosing spondilitis, Reiters disease and idiopathic aortopathy associated with ageing.

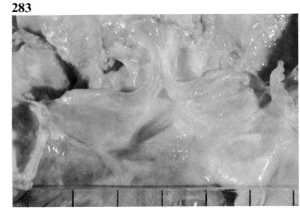

284 Syphilis, aortic valve Superior view to show the degree of incompetence of a syphilitic aortic valve. As in the previous figure there is widening of the commissures and thickening of the upper edges of the cusps, with absence of cusp fusion.

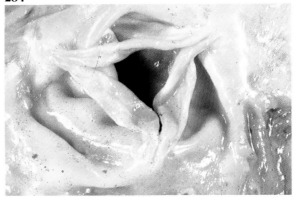

285 Syphilis, aortitis A syphilitic mesoaortitis of the proximal aorta. The intimal surface is wrinkled and puckered with linear wavy depressed scars and thickened white, pearly plaques. This is colloquially described as a 'tree bark' appearance.

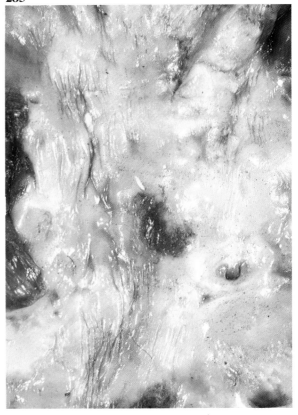

286 Syphilis, aortitis Low power histological appearance of an aorta with syphilitic mesoaortitis. Perivascular cuffing by chronic inflammatory cells is present in a fibrosed adventitia (1) while the media (2) shows disruption of the elastic and muscle with increased vascularisation and surrounding inflammatory cell infiltrate. There is gross fibrous thickening of the intima (3). (*H&E*, ×22)

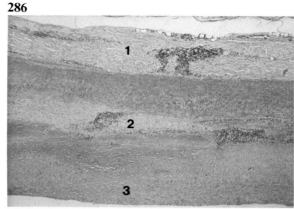

287 Syphilis, aortitis A small artery in the adventitia, with endarteritis obliterans and perivascular cuffing by lymphocytes and plasma cells. (*H&E*, ×140)

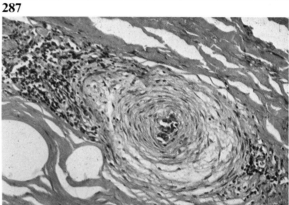

288 Syphilis, aortitis The disruption of the elastic and muscle of the media is more clearly seen in this elastic van Gieson stain. Elastic = stained black. Smooth muscle = brown. Fibrous tissue = red. (*EVG*, ×140)

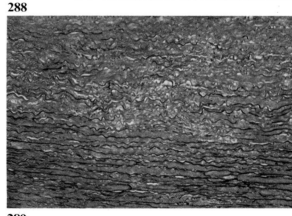

289 Syphilis, aortitis High magnification of thin walled blood vessels in the media surrounded by plasma cells and lymphocytes. (*H&E*, ×352)

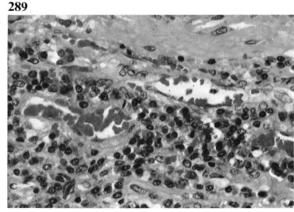

Other valve conditions

A variety of degenerative, ageing and other miscellaneous diseases affecting the valves of the heart are illustrated in this section.

The distinctive shape and appearance of the aortic aspect of the valve is valuable in differentiating the three main causes of aortic stenosis in adults.

290 shows the characteristic transverse slit orifice of calcific aortic stenosis;

291 shows the tri-radiate orifice of senile calcific aortic valve disease;

256 shows the small central triangular orifice seen in severe rheumatic heart disease.

290 Calcific aortic valve disease Superior view of a congenital, bicuspid aortic valve (see **62**) with nodular, calcified masses on the superior surface of the cusps. Calcification of the median raphe (*arrow*) is also present. Note the slit-like orifice. The increased incidence of calcification in this type of valve is due to a greater likelihood of undergoing degenerative changes as a result of 'wear and tear'.

291 Senile calcific aortic valve stenosis A tricuspid aortic valve, viewed from above, with nodular, calcified masses on the aortic side of the cusps. There are no adhesions of the commissures and the free edges of the cusps are not involved. This type of calcification is seen with increasing age and in a small proportion of patients produces aortic stenosis.

292 Mitral valve ring calcification Mitral valve of a heart from a 75-year-old female, distorted by extensive calcification at the valve ring. This condition is seen more commonly with increasing longevity, particularly in women, and often results in mitral incompetence and less commonly in mitral stenosis. It may cause conduction abnormalities, contribute to congestive cardiac failure, and can predispose to endocarditis.

290

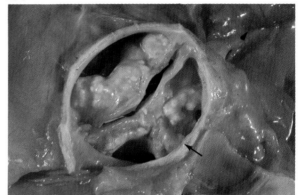

291

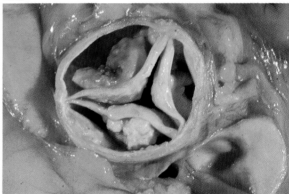

292

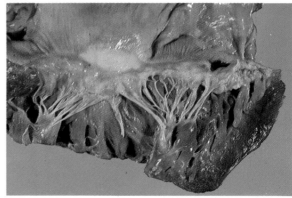

293 Mitral valve ring calcification Posterior leaflet of the mitral valve, shown in the previous figure, lifted up to show a nodular calcified mass at the valve ring. There is no erosion of the cusp endothelium in this heart, a complication which is surprisingly infrequent considering the gross distortion of the leaflet that can be produced by the calcified mass. When erosion does occur super-imposed infective endocarditis or thrombus formation may result (see **312**).

294–296 Mitral valve ring calcification Section across three mitral valves with calcification at the valve ring showing varying appearances of the contents of the mass from pus-like (**294**) to cheesy (**295**) to hard nodular material (**296**). The appearances of **295** should not be confused with a tuberculoma (see **356**) or a gumma.

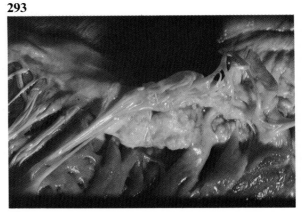

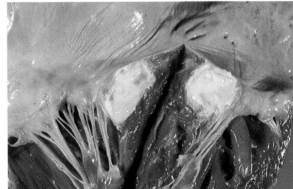

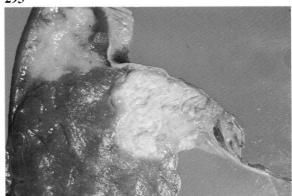

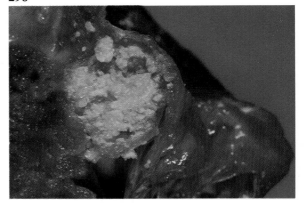

297 Floppy valve Superior view of a floppy mitral valve with ballooning, or doming, of the leaflets. The stretching of the leaflets results from collagen degeneration associated with the presence of acid mucopolysaccharide and softening of the fibrosa layer of the valve cusp. Mitral regurgitation may result from prolapsing of the valve. The aetiology of this condition is obscure but it may possibly have a genetic or age-related background or both.

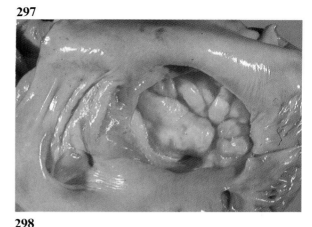

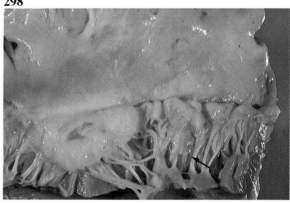

298 Floppy valve The same mitral valve as illustrated in the previous figure opened to show the characteristic ballooning of the leaflets. The mitral valve is the most commonly affected valve with the posterior cusp usually being more severely ballooned than the anterior cusp although in this heart the latter leaflet is the more severely diseased. Also shown is a rare complication of fibrous tethering of chordae tendineae due to friction (*arrow*). The tricuspid valve may also be affected but the changes have little haemodynamic effect. Severe mucoid degeneration of the aortic valve is usually only seen in conditions such as the Marfan syndrome.

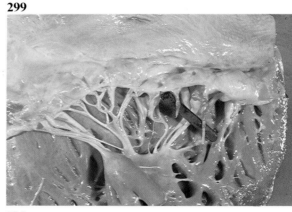

299 Floppy valve with ruptured chordae tendineae An important complication of a floppy valve is rupture of chordae tendineae. It is due to increased tension on the chordae produced by the abnormal movement of the ballooned leaflets. Another complication is infective endocarditis which is illustrated in a later section (see **313**). Rarely sudden death may occur.

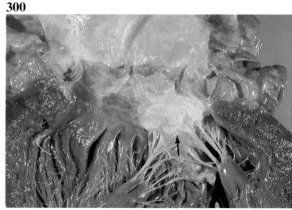

300 Atheroma of mitral valve This anterior cusp of the mitral valve of the heart of an elderly man illustrates that atheromatous deposits (*arrow*) may occur in this valve. They are usually present in the ventricular surface of this cusp with the lipid deposits mainly confined to the fibrosa layer of the valve.

301 Carcinoid heart disease The pulmonary (1) and tricuspid (2) valves of this heart are thickened and contracted due to superimposed fibrosis resulting from a carcinoid syndrome in a 77-year-old female. Note that the chordae tendineae of the tricuspid valve are also affected. These valve lesions occur in patients with metastatic carcinoid tumour, and this heart was from a 77-year-old woman who had a primary carcinoid tumour in the ileum with extensive hepatic metastases. The valves on the left side of the heart are only rarely affected in this condition. The pathogenesis of these changes is uncertain, but is associated with the presence of 5-hydroxytryptamine.

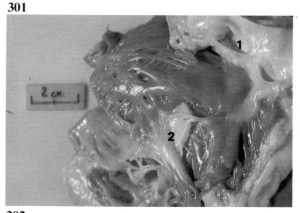

302 Carcinoid heart disease Relatively acellular fibrous tissue (*arrow*), staining rather poorly, covering the surface of an otherwise basically normal tricuspid valve (1). (*H&E,* × 55)

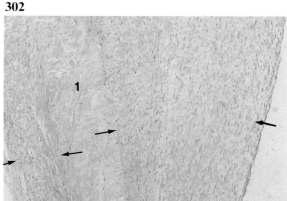

303 Lambl's excrescence A row of filiform excrescences on the contact surface of an aortic valve. These excrescences are thought to be wear and tear lesions and probably develop by thrombus adhering to small tags of torn valve collagen. They are commonly found on the aortic and mitral valves.

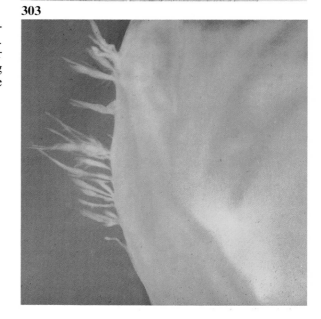

117

304 Lambl's excrescence A small papillary tumour on an aortic valve resembling a 'sea anemone', formed by adhesion of a number of filiform excrescences.

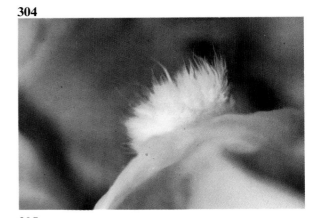

305 Lambl's excrescence These excrescences are also seen on diseased valves as illustrated on this excised rheumatic mitral valve.

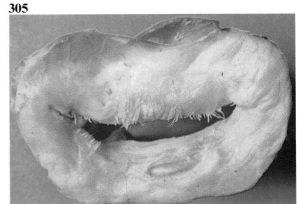

306 Lambl's excrescence Histology shows that these papillary excrescences are composed of avascular hyaline fronds covered by a single layer of epithelium. (*H&E*, × 22)

307 Lambl's excrescence At higher power there is a characteristic granular ring structure which specific stains show to be elastotic. The fronds, however, are probably derived from organising fibrin. (*H&E*, × 88)

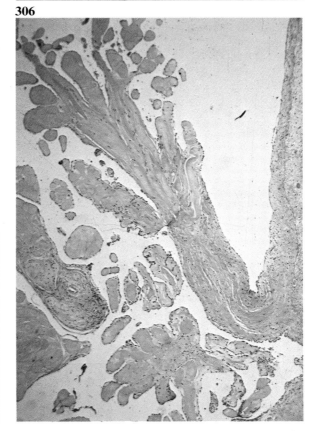

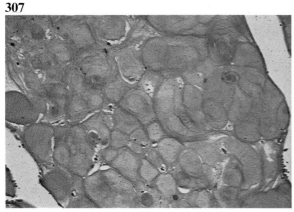

Infective and non-bacterial thrombotic endocarditis

The pattern of infective endocarditis has changed over the last few decades in many countries following the introduction of antibiotics. Whereas it used to predominantly affect young adults with chronic rheumatic heart disease, at the present time it is increasingly seen in elderly patients with normal or degenerative valves. *Streptococcus viridans* still remains an important cause, but there is an increased incidence due to other streptococci, staphylococci, gram-negative bacteria and other organisms. Subdivision pathologically should be based on the causative organism and the pathology, if any, of the valve. The incidence of left sided endocarditis is much greater compared with the right side, due to the higher closing pressure on the left side with consequent increased likelihood of damage to the atrial and mitral valves.

308 Infective endocarditis A vegetation on a mitral valve thickened by rheumatic heart disease. *Streptococcus viridans* was cultured from the vegetation.

308

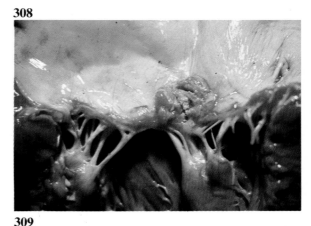

309 Infective endocarditis A large papillary, haemorrhagic vegetation on a mitral valve with mild non-specific post-inflammatory thickening. *Streptococcus faecalis* was isolated following culture of the vegetation.

309

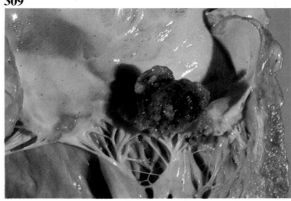

310 Infective endocarditis A cross-section of the valve illustrated in the previous figure showing the degree of cusp thickening and the size of the vegetation.

310

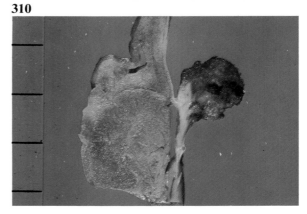

311 Infective endocarditis A staphylococcal aureus endocarditis with perforation of the mitral valve. The remainder of the valve shows only very mild non-specific thickening of the leaflets.

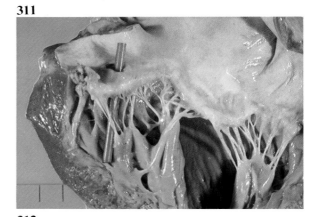

312 Infective endocarditis Infective vegetations present on a mitral valve with ring calcification (see **292**) causing distortion of the leaflets. Pneumococci were cultured from the vegetations.

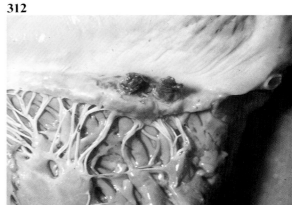

313 Infective endocarditis Infective vegetations (*arrow*) diffusely scattered, mainly on the contact margin, of a moderately 'floppy' ballooned mitral valve (see **297**). A non-haemolytic streptococcus was cultured from these vegetations which probably originated on areas of endothelial damage produced by stretching and excessive folding of the cusps.

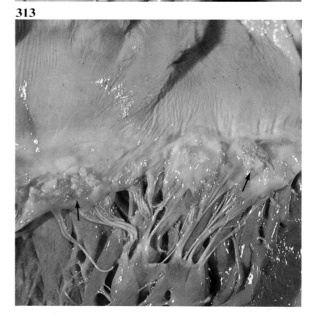

120

314 Infective endocarditis Ruptured chordae tendineae of a mitral valve occurring as a complication of an infective endocarditis.

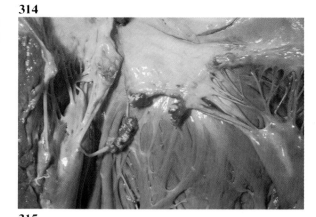

315 Infective endocarditis A staphylococcal aureus endocarditis of the aortic valve. The non-affected portions of the cusps appear normal.

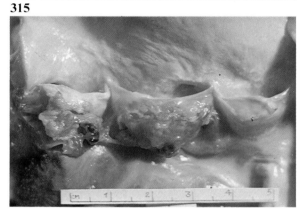

316 Infective endocarditis Extensive ulceration of the aortic valve cusps has occurred in this bacterial endocarditis which failed to respond to antibiotic treatment.

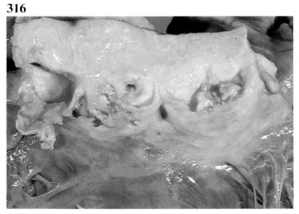

317 Infective endocarditis A florid ulcerating infective endocarditis of the aortic valve with a mural endocarditis also present below the valve. There is an opening of a small aneurysm in the middle of the anterior leaflet of the mitral valve, seen on the right (see **318**).

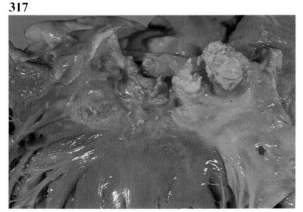

318 Infective endocarditis The aneurysm, described in the previous figure, viewed from the other side of the anterior leaflet of the mitral valve. This aneurysm is probably due to altered haemodynamics resulting from partial destruction of the aortic valve cusps as a consequence of severe endocarditis.

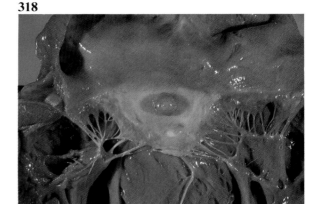

319 Infective endocarditis Infective vegetations almost completely fill a ventricular septal defect (*arrow*) in this infant's heart. In addition a congenital subvalvar aortic fibrous ring extending to the anterior mitral cusp is present below the defect (see **50**).

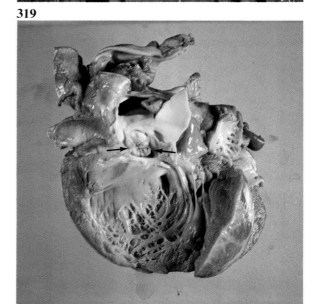

320 Infective endocarditis A florid infective endocarditis is seen on a Starr-Edwards artificial ball valve replacing a mitral valve which was severely affected by rheumatic heart disease.

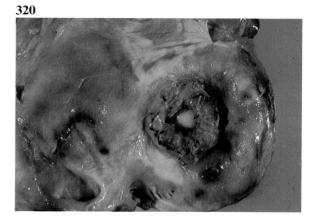

321 Infective endocarditis Close-up of the edge of a fibrosed, vascularised, inflamed rheumatic valve (1) with a dense inflammatory cell infiltrate at the attachment (2) of a vegetation. The latter is composed predominantly of fibrin (3), but contains collections of blue staining cocci (*arrow*). (*H&E*, × 55)

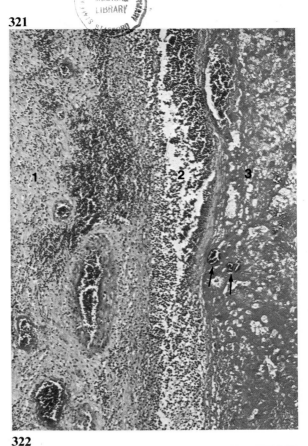

322 & 323 Infective endocarditis Greater detail of an infective vegetation. In **322** inflammatory cells and erythrocytes are shown enmeshed in fibrin, while in **323** numerous blue staining cocci are present, distributed diffusely and in aggregations. (*H&E*, × 140, × 352)

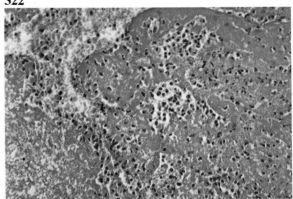

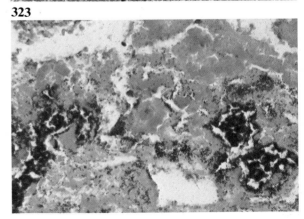

324 Infective endocarditis A large round mass of monilial hyphae is filling the right atrium, while smaller monilial vegetations are present along the tricuspid valve. The heart was from a 17-year-old boy who had had multiple transfusions for aplastic anaemia.

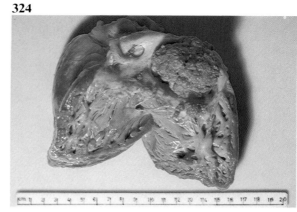

325 Non-bacterial thrombotic endocarditis Two nodular, thrombotic, sterile vegetations on a mitral valve with only mild non-specific thickening of the leaflets. These vegetations, seen mainly on the mitral and aortic valves, are often associated with wasting systemic disease, and in particular with terminal pancreatic and other adenocarcinomas. This is probably now the commonest type of endocarditis, but except for the occurence of emboli this vegetation is usually of no clinical importance. The vegetations may vary in appearance from small to large lesions, be single or multiple and be grossly indistinguishable from infective vegetations. Valve pathology, which may be minor, is often present.

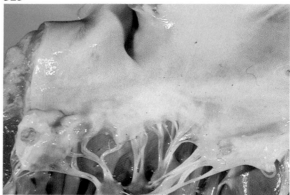

326 Non-bacterial thrombotic endocarditis The vegetation is composed almost entirely of fibrin and there is an absence of inflammatory cells both within the vegetation and the valve (see figures **321–323**). (*H&E*, × 55)

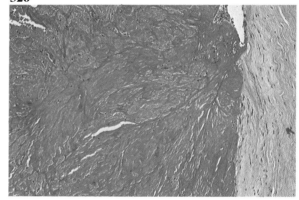

Myocardial degenerations and infiltrations

This section illustrates a selection of ageing, degenerative and infiltrative conditions seen in the myocardium. These processes when seen in the valves are illustrated in the section 'Other valve diseases'.

327 Cloudy swelling One of the first signs of myocardial damage, seen in a wide range of toxic or infective conditions, is swelling of the muscle fibres and granularity of the cytoplasm, known as cloudy swelling. (*H&E*, × 352)

328 Mycocytolysis Vacuolation of myocardial fibres indicates more severe damage than cloudy swelling. This type of degeneration is often known as mycocytolysis and is commonly seen with myocardial ischaemia but can be present in a wide variety of conditions. (*H&E*, × 352)

329 Basophilic degeneration Myocardium with a basophilic mucinous degeneration (*arrow*) of one of the muscle fibres. The cause of this non-specific change is unknown, but it is a common finding at post-mortem, particularly in elderly patients. It may also be associated with myxoedema and primary cardiomyopathy. (*H&E*, × 352)

330 Fragmented fibres Fragmentation, or cracking of myocardial fibres, is probably an artefact occurring in the preparation of the section, particularly from necropsy material. (*H&E*, × 140)

327

328

329

330

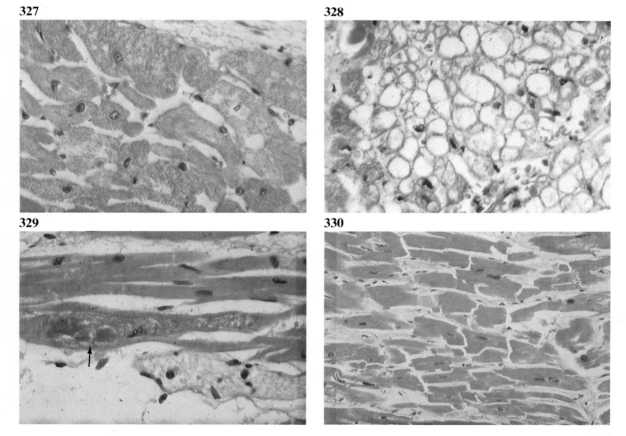

331 Brown atrophy of the heart The opened left ventricle of a small, 125g, heart with brown atrophy of the myocardium. Compare with normal heart. Although not illustrated, the main coronary arteries are characteristically tortuous in this condition.

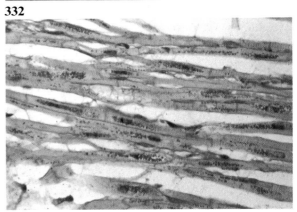

332 Brown atrophy of the heart Lipofuscin, probably derived from lysosomal contents, is found universally in the elderly. Brown atrophy means coincidental pigment accumulation and cardiac atrophy such as occurs in a wasting disease. This figure shows lipofuscin granules, particularly located at the nuclear poles of atrophic myocardial fibres, coloured red on a PAS stain. In H&E stains these granules appear yellow-brown. (*PAS,* × 550)

333 Fatty degeneration Pale flecks are scattered throughout the myocardium of this left ventricle. This is colloquially known as 'tabby-cat' or 'thrush breast' appearance and is due to fatty degeneration of the myocardial muscle fibres. This heart is from a patient who had longstanding severe anaemia and the distribution of fat is mainly subendocardial. A more diffuse fatty degeneration is seen in toxaemic deaths and in many other diseases.

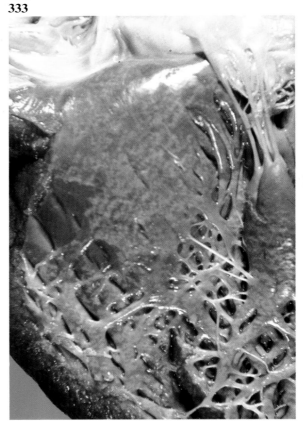

334 Fatty degeneration Cross-sections of myo-cardial fibres showing the distribution of small fatty droplets within the fibres. (*SUDAN III*, × 334)

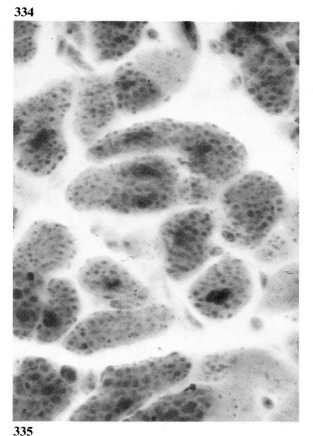

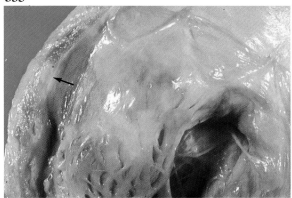

335 Fatty infiltration (cardiac adiposity) Extensive fatty infiltration of the right ventricular wall in the pulmonary outflow tract. In one portion of the wall the muscle appears to be almost completely absent (*arrow*). This condition usually affects the right ventricle more severely than the other chambers and is occasionally responsible for right ventricular failure.

336 Fatty infiltration (cardiac adiposity) Extensive adipose tissue extending among atrophic myo-cardial fibres of the right ventricle. (*H&E*, × 55)

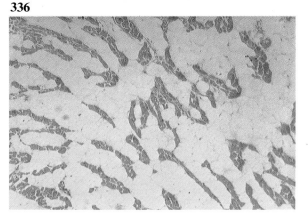

337 Myocardial calcification Numerous, ill-defined, calcified areas in the myocardium of a hypertrophied left ventricle. The cause of this unusually extensive calcification remained uncertain but was probably post-infective and dystrophic in type. The heart was from a young male adult with no evidence of coronary artery disease. The commonest type of dystrophic calcification, however, is in ventricular aneurysms, following myocardial infarction, particularly in elderly men.

337

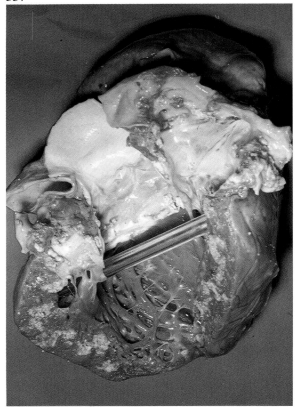

338 Myocardial calcification An x-ray of the heart illustrated in the previous figure shows more clearly the extent of the calcification of the myocardium.

338

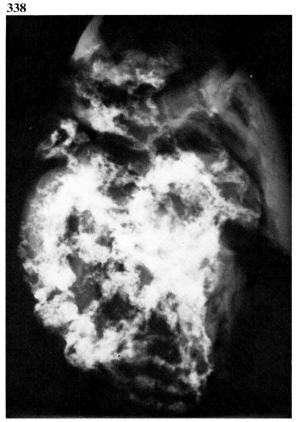

339 Myocardial calcification Metastatic calcification of myocardial fibres with adjacent normal fibres. The heart was from a 51-year-old female who had hypercalcaemia. (*H&E,* ×140)

339

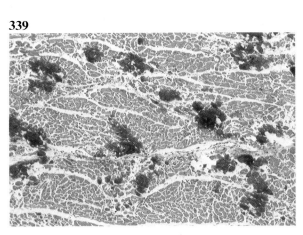

340 Haemochromatosis Myocardial fibres severely damaged by deposition of iron with resulting extensive fibrosis. These appearances may be seen in patients with either haemochromatosis or haemosiderosis. Grossly, the heart is usually enlarged and brown in colour. Acid ferrocyanide application results in a blue-green colour. Congestive cardiac failure occurs when myocardial damage is severe. (*H&E*, × 140)

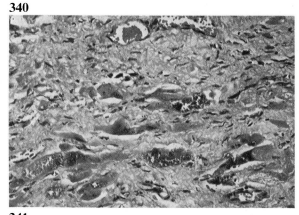

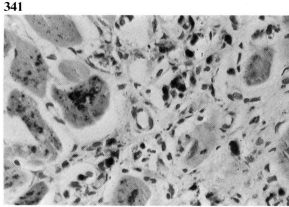

341 Haemochromatosis A Perl's stain of the same section illustrated in the previous figure shows more clearly the heavy deposition of iron (staining blue) in the myocardial fibres, in the surrounding macrophages, and interstitial tissue. (× 352)

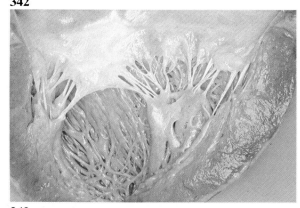

342 Amyloid The pale, waxy appearance of the myocardium of this left ventricle is due to generalised infiltration by amyloid. The heart was from a patient with systemic amyloidosis.

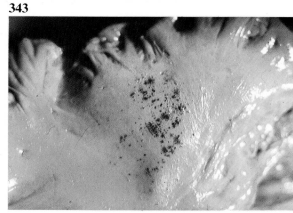

343 Amyloid Close-up of the endocardium of a left atrium with areas of amyloid stained brown-black following the application of Lugol's iodine. This is an example of senile amyloid which is common in patients over 70 years. In approximately three-quarters of the cases the deposition is scanty and confined to the atria, but with extensive deposition cardiac failure may result.

344 Amyloid Section of left ventricle in which there is extensive replacement of the normal muscle fibre structure by amyloid which appears as a hyaline acellular substance lacking any specific features. (*H&E*, × 550)

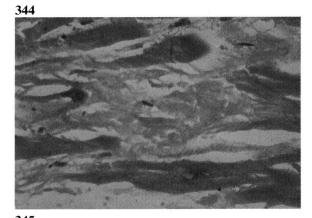

345–347 Amyloid The presence and distribution of amyloid is usually confirmed by special staining techniques. Examples are shown here.

In **345** metachromatic reddish-purple staining amyloid replacing myocardial fibres demonstrated by a crystal violet stain. (× 220)

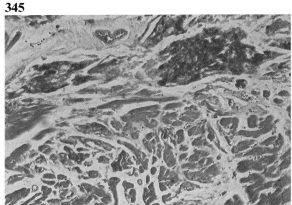

In **346** the presence of amyloid in an aortic valve confirmed by green-orange birefringence with the Congo-red staining method when viewed with the polarising microscope. This is a section of a heart from a patient with secondary amyloidosis associated with longstanding rheumatoid arthritis. (× 550)

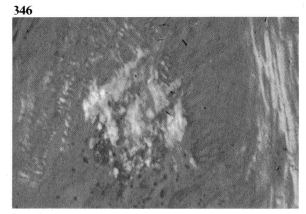

In **347** the amyloid, which is stained green using Lendrum's SAB-van Gieson method, has a typical perifibre distribution in a heart with senile amyloid. (× 352)

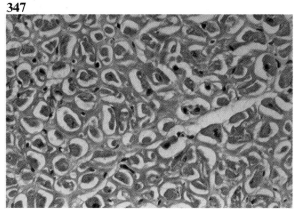

130

Myocarditis

Myocarditis is an inflammatory process of the heart muscle caused by known or unknown agents, but excluding atheromatous coronary artery disease. Aetiological agents which have so far been recognised include specific or non-specific infective organisms, chemicals, physical agents, drugs, and hypersensitivity reactions.

In this section, examples of myocarditis due mainly to infectious agents are illustrated.

348 Pyaemic abscesses A museum specimen with small pyaemic abscesses in the outer part of the wall of the left ventricle of a heart of a boy aged 9 years. The abscesses developed following acute osteomyelitis of the left femur.

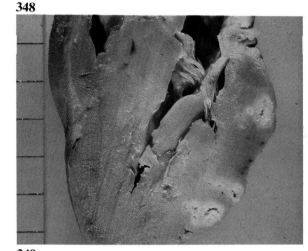

349 Acute bacterial myocarditis An area of acute inflammation with early muscle necrosis and two collections of dark blue staining staphylococci. This type of inflammation may accompany a septicaemia. (*H&E*, × 88)

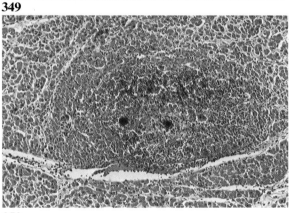

350 Pyaemic abscess A small pyaemic abscess in the myocardium. An oval area of myocardium has been destroyed and is replaced by a collection of dark blue staining polymorphonuclear leucocytes. In the centre of the abscess there is a collection of bacteria appearing as a small darker blue blob. (*H&E*, × 55)

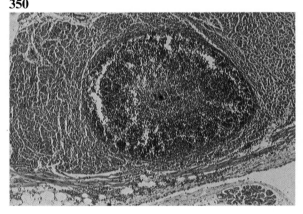

131

351 Viral myocarditis An acute Coxsackie B viral myocarditis with a dense inflammatory cell infiltrate, predominantly mononuclear in type, related to degenerate myocardial fibres. (*H&E*, ×704)

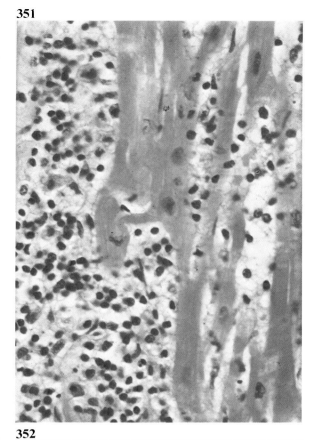

352 Idiopathic myocarditis A focal area of degenerate myocardial fibres with a surrounding inflammatory cell infiltrate consisting predominantly of lymphocytes, but with scattered neutrophils and eosinophils. (*H&E*, ×704)

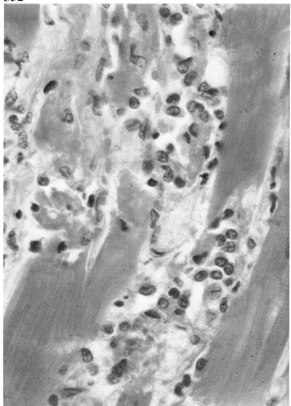

353

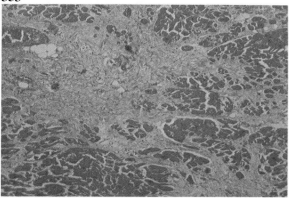

353 Healed myocarditis A fibrous scar in the myocardium formed following a viral myocarditis. (*H&E*, ×55)

354 Giant cell myocarditis Well defined semitranslucent grey areas of myocardial damage, with a surrounding rim of whitish myocardium, characteristic of a giant cell myocarditis.

355 Giant cell myocarditis A diffuse, severe myocarditis with fairly numerous giant cells. These latter cells are of myogenic origin, but the aetiology of the condition is unknown. (*H&E*, ×280)

354

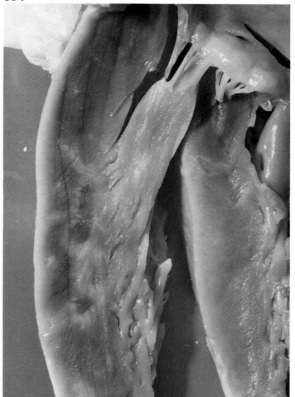

355

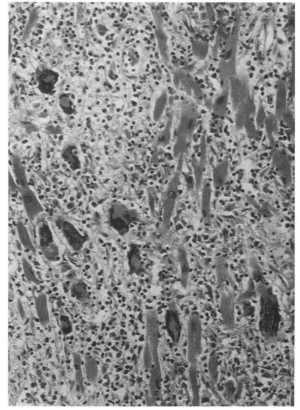

356 Tuberculosis An opened left ventricle with a caseating tuberculoma in the upper interventricular septum. The appearances should not be confused with the cheese-like masses sometimes present in mitral valve ring calcification (see **295**).

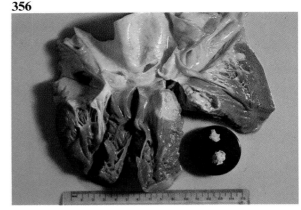

357 Tuberculosis Granulomata, consisting of a small central area of caseation surrounded by histiocytes, scanty lymphocytes and Langhan's type giant cells, within the myocardium. (*H&E*, × 140)

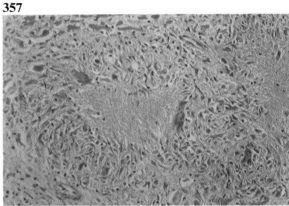

358 Sarcoidosis The myocardium may be focally or diffusely involved in about a fifth of patients with this systemic, granulomatous condition of unknown aetiology. The sarcoid granulomata consist of a collection of histiocytes with surrounding scanty lymphocytes and occasional giant cells scattered within the myocardium. In contrast to tuberculosis there is no central caseation. (*H&E,* × 140)

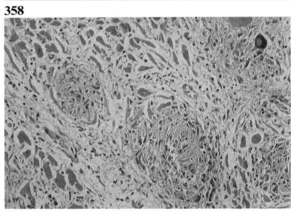

359 Protozoal myocarditis Cysts filled with *Toxoplasma gondii*, as illustrated here, are only rarely found within the myocardial fibres of human hearts. This heart showed a severe myocarditis with a mixed inflammatory cell infiltrate. (*H&E,* × 550)

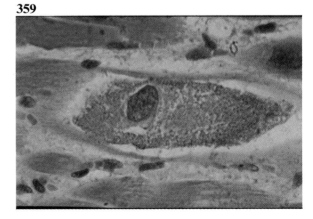

360 Protozoal myocarditis Colonies of *Trypanosoma cruzi* present within a myocardial fibre. This type of myocarditis, known as Chagas' disease, is most commonly seen in South America where the protozoal organism is widespread. In this myocarditis the mainly chronic inflammatory cell infiltrate related to degenerate myocardial fibres probably results from release of parasites from the pseudocysts of *Trypanosoma cruzi*. (*H&E,* ×550)

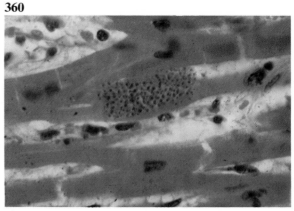

361 Myocarditis, cysticercus cellulosae Scattered small cysts (*arrow*) of *C. cellulosae* are protruding from the epicardial surface of the left ventricle. This is the larval stage of a *Taenia Solium* infestation.

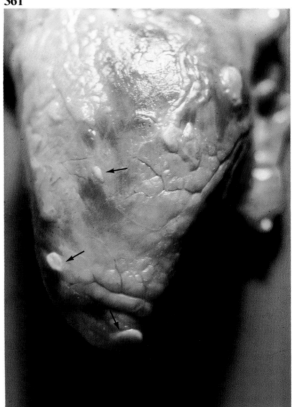

362 Myocarditis, cysticercus cellulosae Lying within the myocardium is seen a cyst containing a cross-section of the worm with the scolex in the centre. (*H&E,* ×8.8)

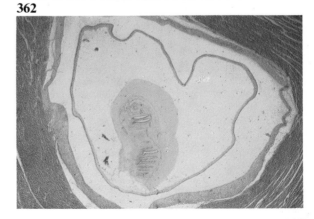

Familial diseases

A few examples of genetically determined diseases are illustrated in this section.

363 Muscular dystrophy The opened left ventricle of a heart from a 24-year-old male with muscular dystrophy of the pseudo-hypertrophic type. The wall is thin due to fibrous replacement of the myocardium which is most easily seen in the middle and inner part of the cut wall (*arrow*).

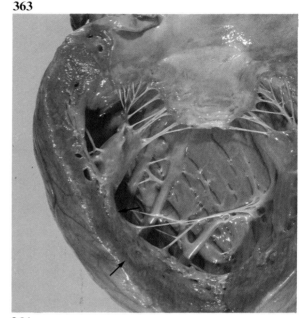

364 Muscular dystrophy Histology of the heart in the previous figure shows extensive diffuse, fibrous tissue surrounding isolated and small groups of atypical muscle fibres. (*H&E,* × 220)

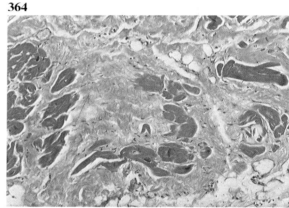

365 Glycogen storage disease Characteristic lace-like appearances of the muscle fibres which in life were distended with large amounts of glycogen. The heart was from a child of 8 months who had a familial type II (Pompe) glycogen storage disease. Extreme cardiomegaly is characteristic of this condition. (*H&E,* × 140)

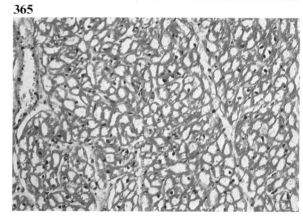

370 Sino-atrial node The sino-atrial node (*arrow*) is situated just below the summit of the right atrium at its junction with the superior vena cava (1). The crest of the atrial appendage (2) is a useful marker of the position of the node. The node is normally crescentic in shape being approximately 15 × 15 × 1.5mm in size and lies with its long axis along the sino-atrial junction. The node is most easily located histologically by excising the entire sino-atrial junction and then cutting longitudinal blocks for sectioning. Before this is done the heart should have been fixed in formalin after lightly packing the superior vena cava with cotton wool to retain its shape. 3 = pulmonary valve; 4 = aortic valve.

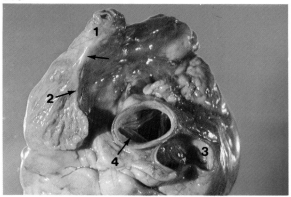

371 The sino-atrial node The node (1) is located around the sino-atrial node artery (2) adjacent to the fatty epicardium. It consists of a network arrangement of small, poorly striated myofibres lying within a dense fibrous connective tissue. The specialised role of the nodal tissue is to initiate impulses whereas the bundle branches allow rapid conduction of these impulses. This sino-atrial node, from a 60-year-old, shows a slight increase in adipose tissue at the periphery of the node, occurring as an ageing process. (*H&E*, × 140)

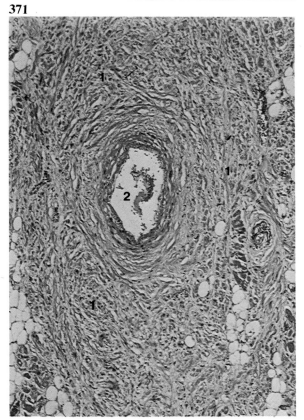

372 The conduction system in the ventricles This is examined from the right ventricle. The atrio-ventricular node (1) lies between the opening of the coronary sinus (2) and the medial leaflet of the tricuspid valve. The approximate path of the atrio-ventricular bundle (3) and right bundle branch (4) is drawn here.

Excision of the atrio-ventricular node and ventricular conduction system for histological study may be carried out by cutting two blocks from the septum as illustrated. The initial cut is the most important and is made vertically into the septum immediately anterior to the coronary sinus. The other vertical cut must be sufficiently anterior to include all the membranous septum. The upper horizontal cut should be about 0.5cm above this membranous septum. The lower horizontal cuts are made so that the upper block contains the atrio-ventricular node and origin of the bundle branches and the lower block contains the distal portions of the bundle branches. The latter block should later be sectioned in the horizontal plane and the former block in the vertical plane. Following processing the blocks are ideally serially sectioned, but this involves considerable labour. For routine purposes only selected sections are generally studied by pathologists.

372

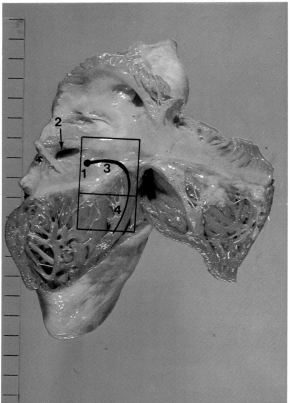

373 Atrio-ventricular node The node (*arrow*) lies beneath the right atrial endocardium and adjacent to the central fibrous body (1) of the heart, which separates the node from the upper septal myocardium. The insertion of the tricuspid valve is just below the node. In contrast to the sino-atrial node there is no large central artery although a small artery and veins are present. (*H&E,* × 55)

373

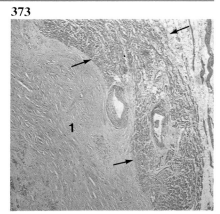

374 Atrio-ventricular node The node consists of loosely interweaving small specialised muscle fibres with strands of connective tissue between them. This higher power shows a superficial portion of parallel arranged fibres that probably connect with atrial conduction fibres, and a deep portion of a network of muscle fibres that gives rise to the main atrio-ventricular bundle. Black radio-opaque injection medium is present within the small blood vessels. (*H&E,* × 88)

374

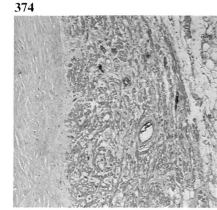

375 Atrio-ventricular bundle, penetrating portion
The conduction fibres from the atrio-ventricular
node pass into the central fibrous body where they
are known as the penetrating portion of the atrio-
ventricular bundle (*arrow*). The bundle is more
condensed than the node and is subdivided by
connective tissue septa with the fibres arranged in
parallel. (*H&E,* × 55)

376 Atrio-ventricular bundle, branching portion
The penetrating portion of the atrio-ventricular
bundle is short and soon gives off the first of the
fascicles of the left bundle branch. As it does so, the
bundle becomes the branching portion. The right
bundle branch (1) is best considered to be the direct
continuation of the main atrio-ventricular bundle
and begins as the last of the fascicles of the left
bundle branch is given off (2) as illustrated here.
(*H&E,* × 55)

377 & 378 Ageing changes in the conduction system
377 Fibrous tissue may increase with age in the
upper part of the muscular interventricular septum
with the collagen often showing focal calcification
(*arrow*). (*H&E,* × 55)
378 Loss of conduction fibres at the origin of the
fascicles of the left bundle branch (*arrow*), is very
commonly associated with the increasing fibrosis
illustrated in the previous figure. (*H&E,* × 88)

Other ageing changes occurring in the conduction system include an increase in adipose and
fibrous tissue in the sino-atrial node and slight
fibrosis in the more distal portion of the left bundle
branch.

375

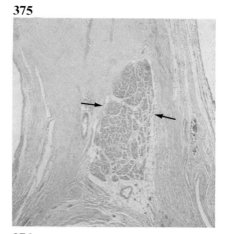

376

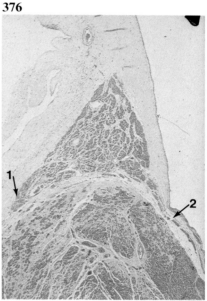

378

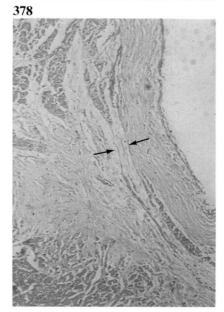

377

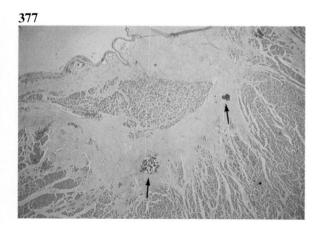

379 Congenital hearts In some congenital malformations of the heart the pathway of the conduction system is altered but still lies in the expected anatomical position if the development of the defect is considered. For example, illustrated here is a ventricular septal defect where the atrioventricular bundle ran in the lower rim of the defect. On the other hand in other congenital malformations, such as corrected transposition, the conduction system is grossly abnormal.

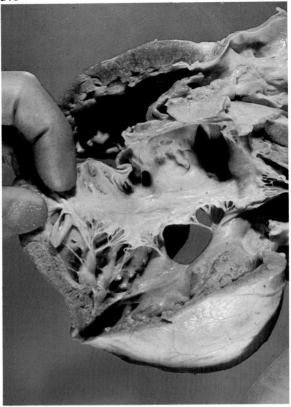

380 Idiopathic bundle branch fibrosis is the commonest cause of complete atrio-ventricular heart block. The histological appearance of one type is illustrated here with a loss of conduction fibres (*arrow*) in a segment of the left bundle branch. The other sites that may be affected are the origin of the left bundle branch plus either fibrosis in the adjacent main bundle or in the right bundle branch. Other important but less frequent causes of complete heart block are ischaemic heart disease, idiopathic congestive cardiomyopathy and calcific valve disease. (*H&E,* ×176)

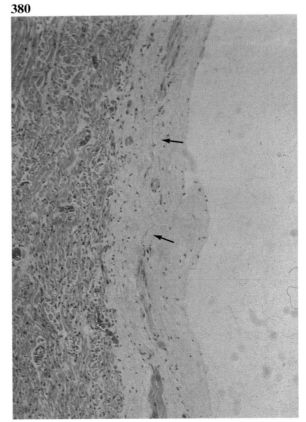

381

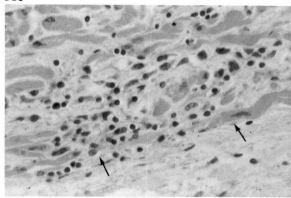

The conduction system may be affected by a variety of diseases involving the heart generally. A few examples are illustrated.

381 A chronic inflammatory cell infiltrate is present in the atrio-ventricular bundle of a heart with diffuse idiopathic myocarditis. (*H&E*, ×550)

382 Granulomatous inflammation of rheumatoid arthritis has destroyed a left bundle branch (*arrow*). (*H&E*, ×280)

383 Metastatic malignant tumour The function of the atrio-ventricular conduction system may be affected by metastatic malignant tumours. Illustrated here is a close-up of the penetrating portion of the atrio-ventricular bundle (*arrow*) infiltrated by a lymphosarcoma. (*H&E*, ×280)

384 Haemorrhage in atrio-ventricular bundle The atrio-ventricular conduction system may occasionally be damaged during cardiac surgery. This figure shows considerable haemorrhage in the branching portion of the atrio-ventricular bundle (1). The haemorrhage was also present around the left bundle branches. (*H&E*, ×55)

383

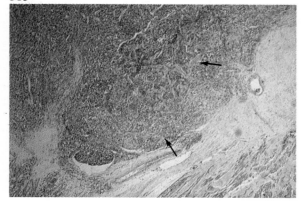

382

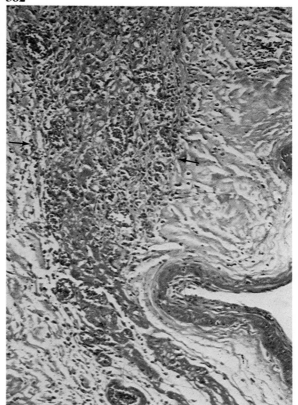

384

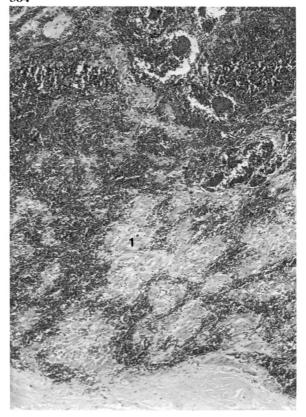

Tumours of the heart

Primary tumours of the heart are rare, with the commonest being myxomas, followed by the group of primary sarcomas. Secondary tumours are much more frequent, with carcinoma of the breast, bronchial carcinoma, malignant melanomas and lymphomas having a relatively high incidence of cardiac involvement.

385 Myxoma of the heart A lobulated myxoma, arising from the interatrial septal wall of the left atrium, extending down partially to occlude the mitral valve opening. This is the commonest site of origin of this benign tumour which although rare is the most frequent primary heart tumour. These tumours should be differentiated from thrombi in the left atrium (see **408**).

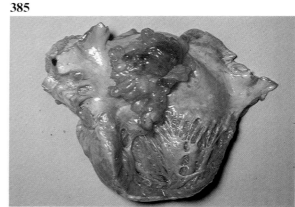

385

386 Myxoma of the heart A myxoma consisting of weakly eosinophilic and basophilic matrix containing scattered stellate and lipidic cells, fibrocytes, occasional blood vessels and scanty haemorrhage. The surface is covered by endothelium. (*H&E*, ×88)

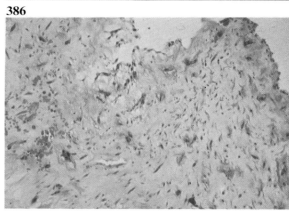

386

387 Fibroma of the heart A large, white, benign fibroma involving the junction of the anterior wall of the left ventricle (1) and interventricular septum (2). The apex of the heart has been cut off and the ventricles are viewed from below. This is a very rare tumour as are other benign cardiac tumours.

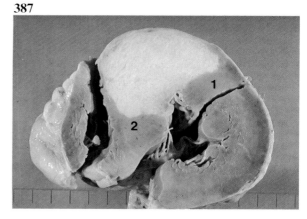

387

388 Fibroma of the heart The edge of a fibroma merging with myocardium on the left. This benign tumour consists of densely packed mature fibroblasts arranged in a slight wavy pattern. Fibrous tissue = blue. Myocardium = red. (*MSB*, × 55)

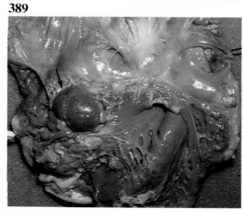

389 Rhabdomyosarcoma of the heart A lobulated and nodular rhabdomyosarcoma (*arrow*) infiltrating the right ventricle of a heart of a 6-year-old child. Primary sarcomas are collectively the second most common primary tumours of the heart after myxomas.

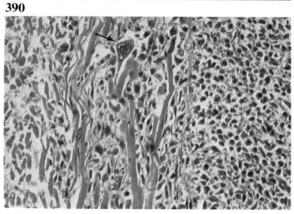

390 & 391 Rhabdomyosarcoma Invasion of myocardium by a rhabdomyosarcoma. The cells vary in shape and size with typical 'strap-like' and 'tennis racquet' cells (*arrow*) being present. (*H&E*, × 140, × 352)

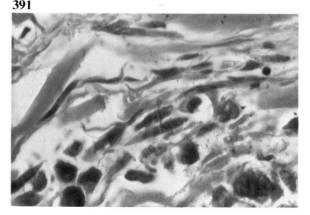

145

392 Myxosarcoma of the heart A museum specimen of a large primary myxosarcoma of the heart involving the apex of the left ventricle.

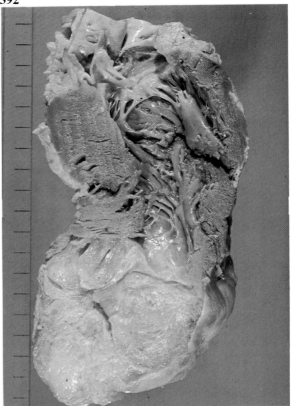

393 Secondary malignant tumour Secondary malignant tumours are considerably more common than primary tumours of the heart. This heart shows a solitary small grey-white nodule of secondary carcinoma invading the myocardium of the left ventricle. The primary tumour was a carcinoma of the breast.

394 Secondary malignant tumour The extent to which the heart may be infiltrated by tumour is shown in this transverse ventricular myocardial slice. The right ventricular wall is almost completely replaced with obliteration of the cavity (1). The primary carcinoma arose in the colon.

394

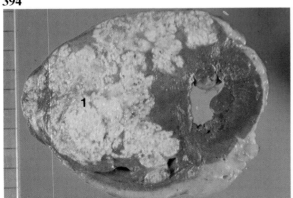

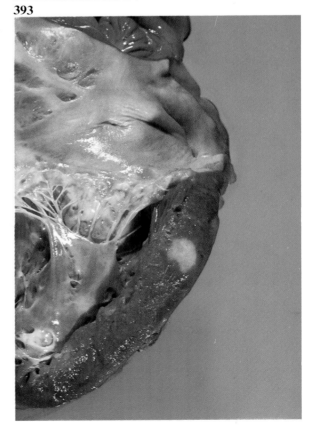

395 Secondary malignant tumour The opened right atrium and ventricle of this heart shows invasion by multiple yellowish deposits of a malignant lymphoma.

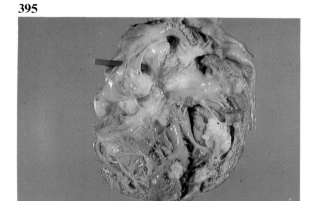

396 Secondary malignant tumour The right ventricle of this heart was diffusely infiltrated by malignant lymphoma and death was due to rupture of the wall.

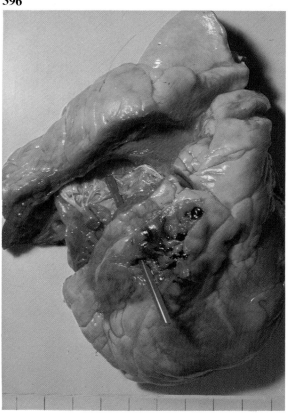

397 Secondary malignant tumour A small nodule of secondary fibrosarcoma protruding from the wall of the auricular appendage of the right atrium.

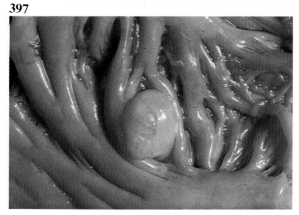

398–402 Secondary malignant tumour These five figures illustrate microscopical appearances of myocardium invaded by secondary malignant tumours of the following types:

398 A mucous producing adenocarcinoma. (*H&E,* ×55)

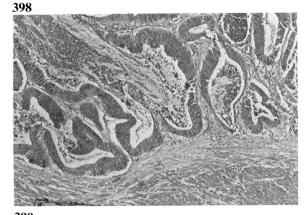

399 A poorly differentiated squamous cell carcinoma. (*H&E,* ×140)

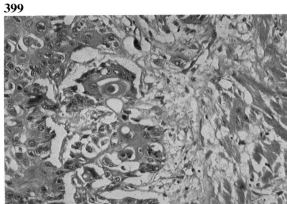

400 A malignant melanoma with brown pigment present in the tumour cells. (*H&E,* ×140)

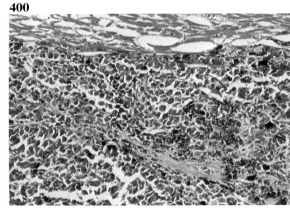

401 A fibrosarcoma. (*H&E,* ×140)
402 A malignant lymphoma. (*H&E,* ×550)

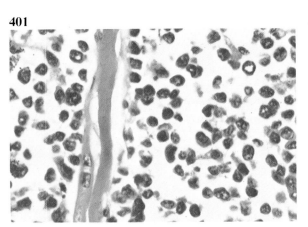

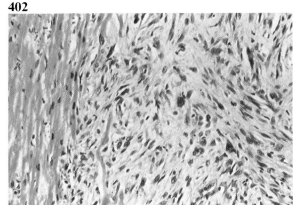